The Little Lion with the BIG ROAR!

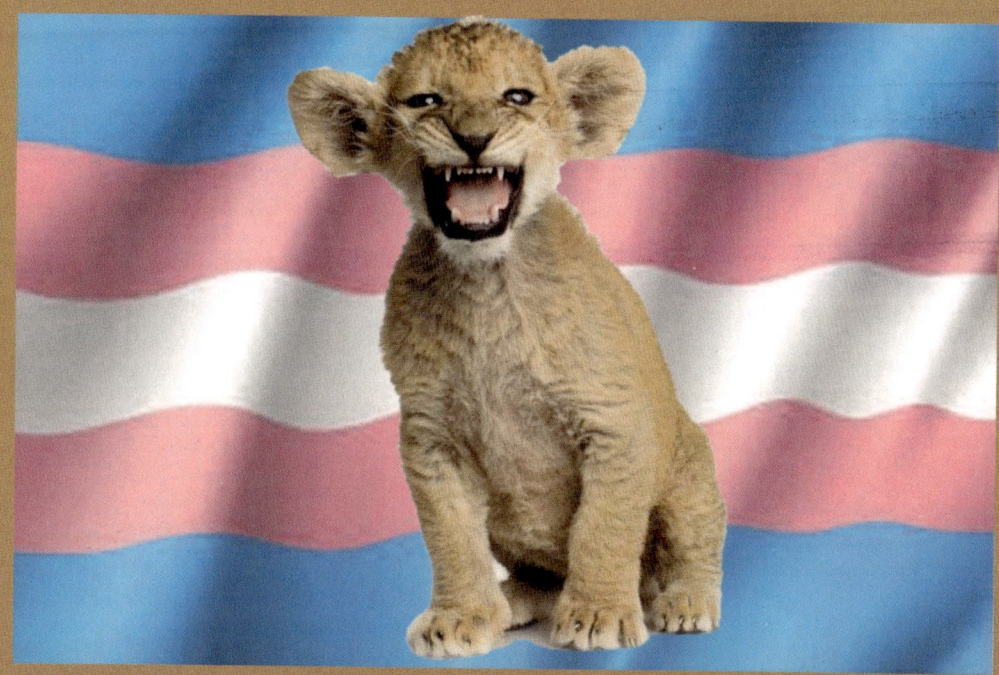

LGBTQ

Elisabeth Broen
2019

Author:
Elisabeth Brown 2019

©elisabethbrown2019
No part of this book maybe reproduced, or stored in a retrieval system in any form, or by any means including electronically, mechanically, recording or otherwise without written permission from Elisabeth Brown:
elisabethbrown13@gmail.com

You don't have to be the biggest, bravest,

King of the Jungle to make the

loudest Roar.

You just have to be the

Proudest Lion

in the Pride

to make an

Impact!

My name is Dillion, which means a male lion.

I am a male lion cub, and I was born into a group of lions called a Pride. There are 15 lions in our Pride.

My Mother, along with other lionesses. There are also four large male lions, one of which is my Father, and there are several other cubs in our pride, besides me.

I have a brother, but no sisters.

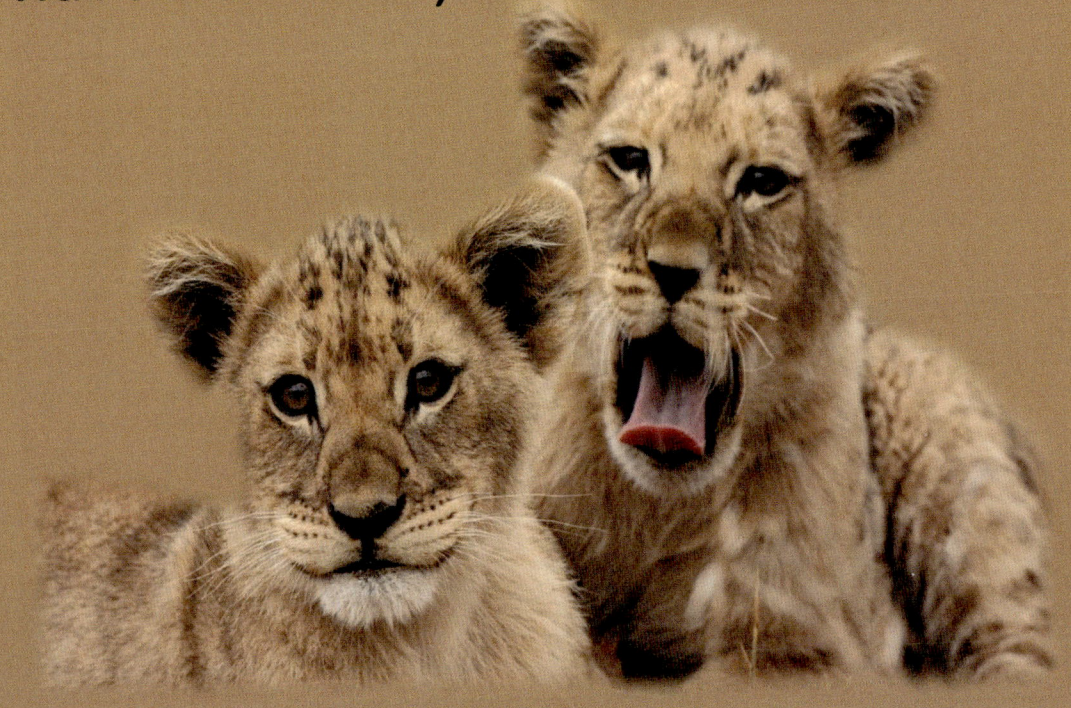

As I grew older, I started to have feelings that I didn't quite understand.

I stayed away from the other cubs and played mostly by myself.

I felt that I was different than the other cubs.

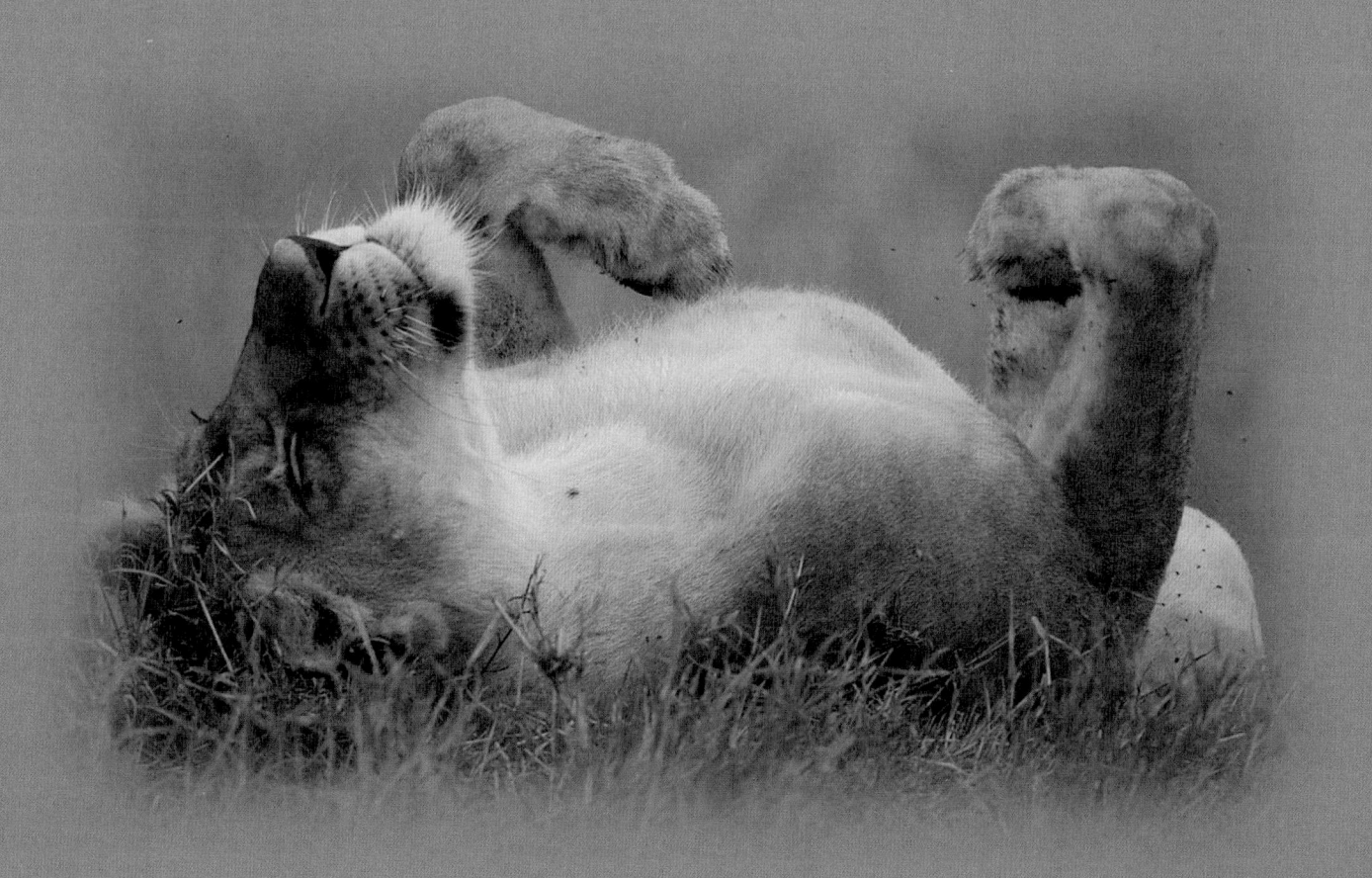

The other male cubs were always rough with each other, jumping, wrestling, and chasing each other around. Always trying to see who was the strongest, or who could roar the loudest, or get the dirtiest.

I didn't really like being around the other male cubs. I didn't understand why, because I was a male cub myself.

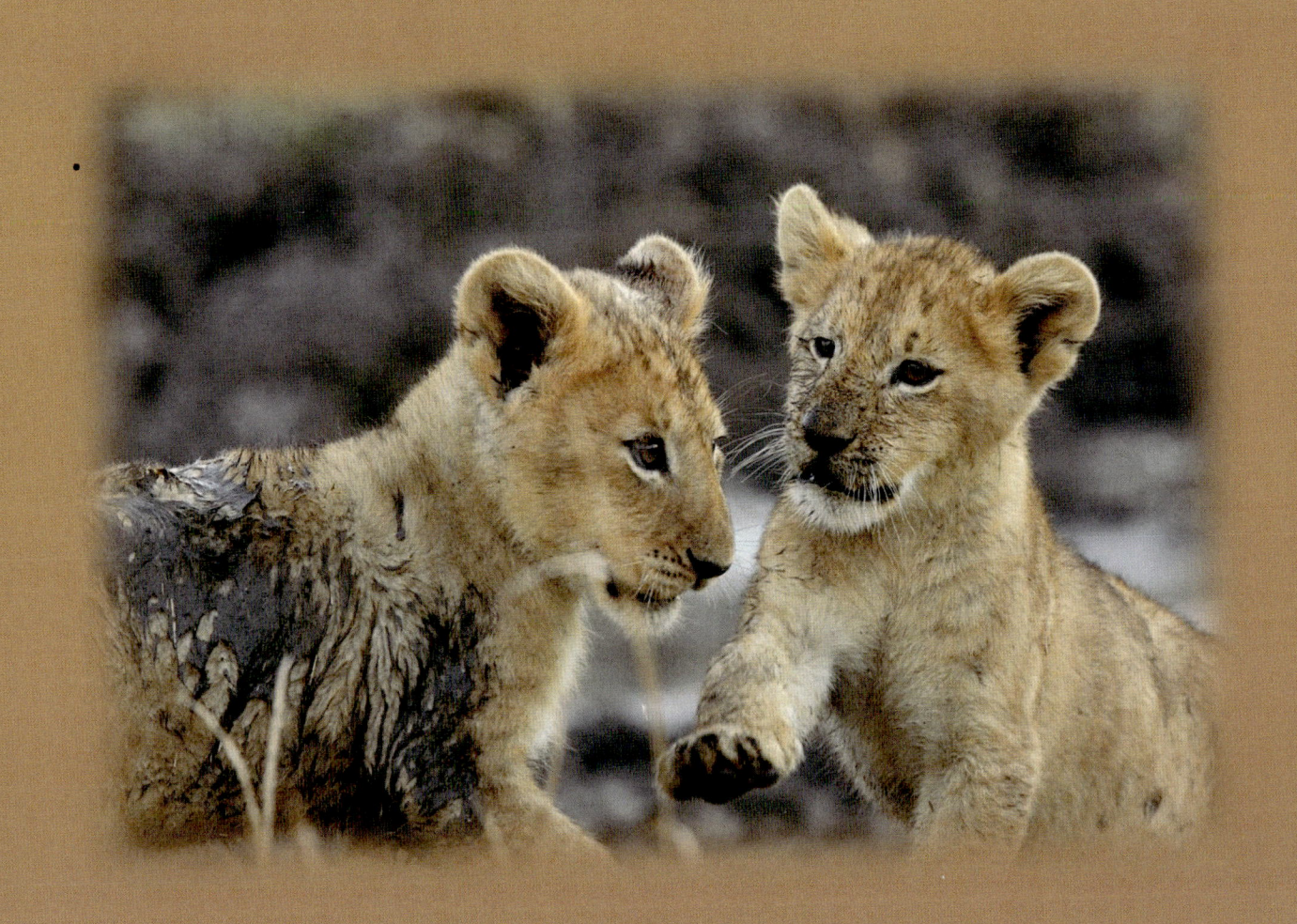

I didn't like those games. I would sit and watch the female cubs play. They always seemed gentler, always cleaning themselves, and making sure that they looked beautiful. They would help their Mothers with bathing the younger cubs. Always making sure everyone was close by, and that they were always well groomed.

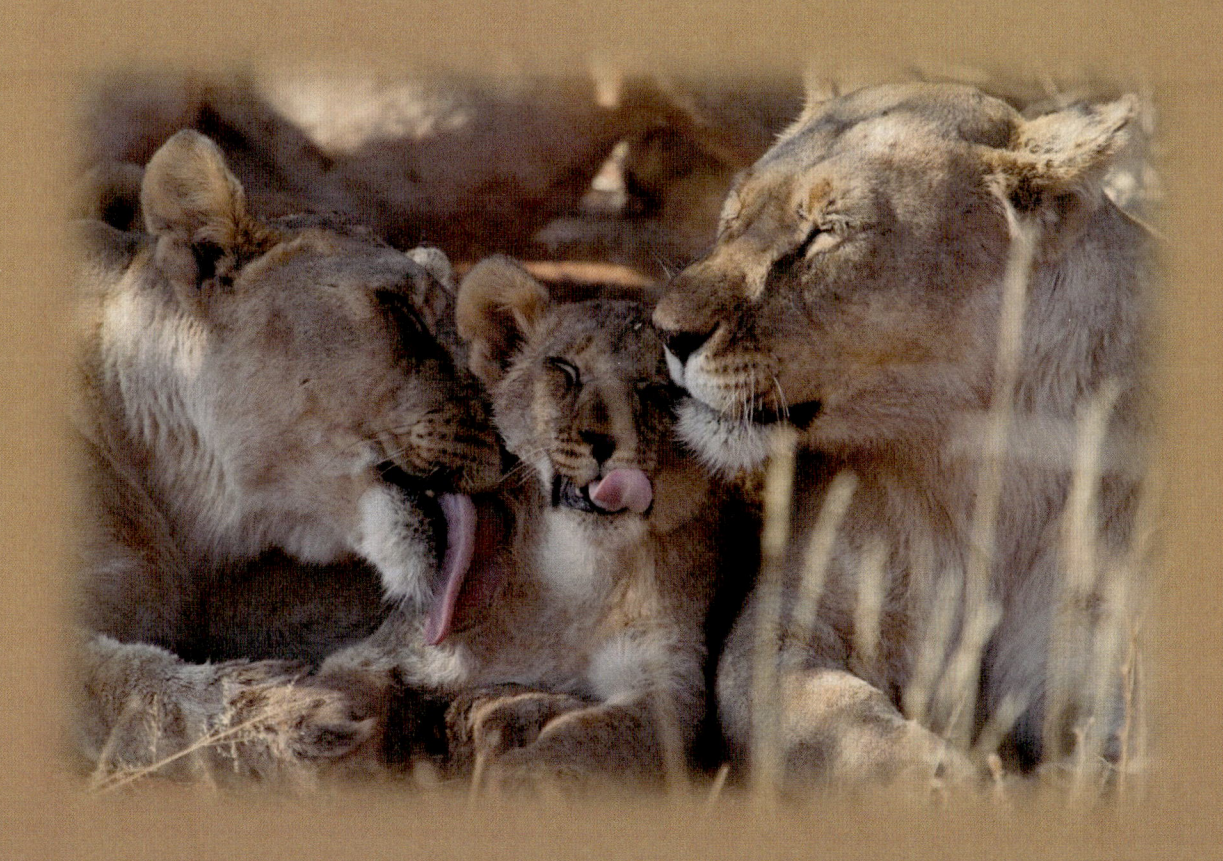

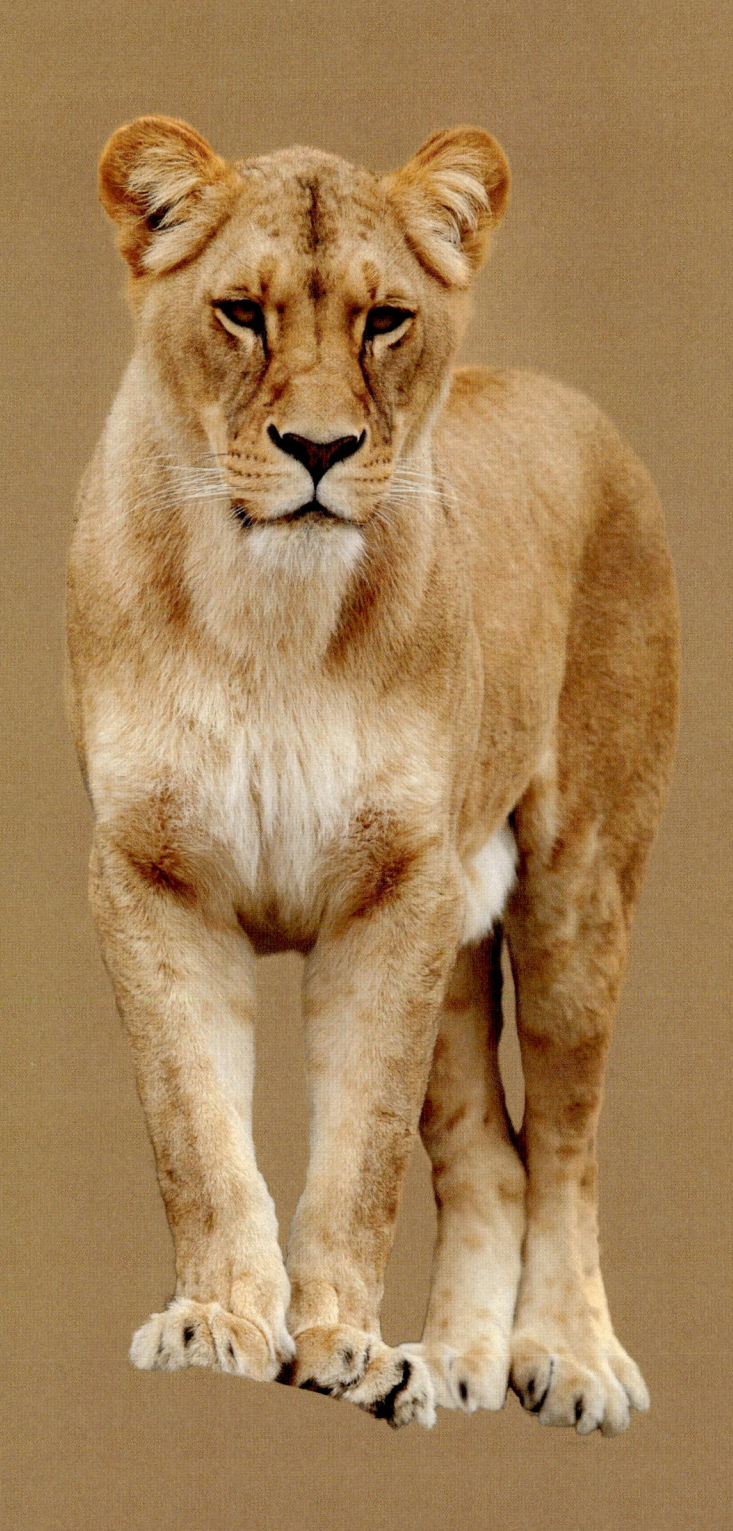

I used to look at my Mother, and think to myself how beautiful she was. If I was a female lion, that is just how I would like to look.

Standing straight, and tall and proud!

The way I had always pictured myself.

I came close to asking my Mother why I felt so different than the other male cubs.

I wanted to tell her, but I felt that no one would accept me, my family or my friends. I thought that others would not understand how I felt.

I thought they would make fun of me, or pick on me. I didn't want any of those things to happen to me or my family.

So, I just continued to hide my inner feelings.

I just went on enjoying the love my own Mother was showing me as her cub, but never got up the nerve to ask her why I felt this way.

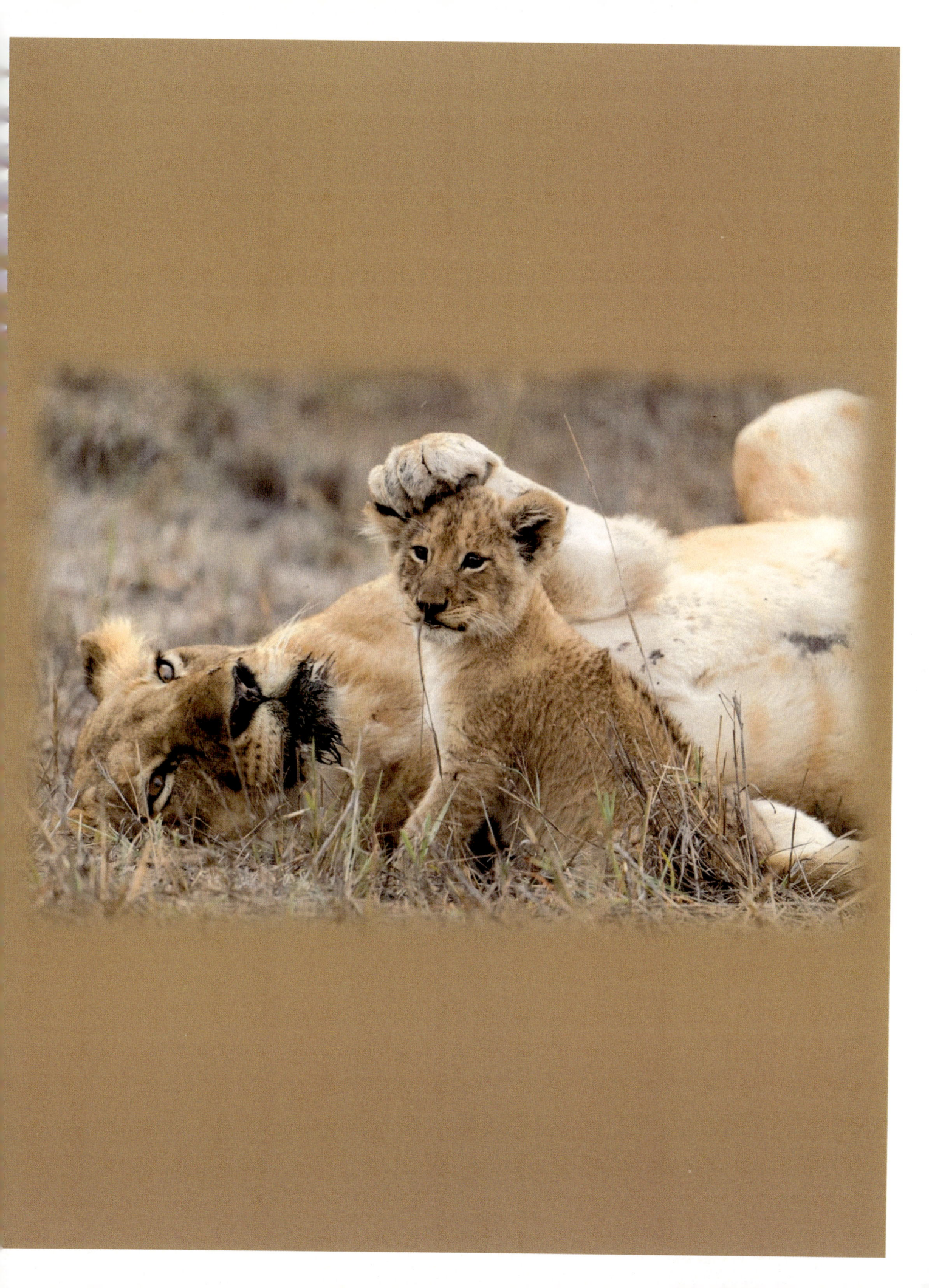

Over the years, I didn't think that anyone else noticed the way that I felt, but they did.

A lot of times when we got together with my family or as a group, I was moody, and didn't want to go. If I did go, I was miserable, but no one ever asked me why.

I wasn't quite sure how to tell any of them. I was afraid that they wouldn't love me or accept me, as the lioness that I really wanted to be.

So, I always said, "I'm tired", or "I don't feel well" or any other excuse that I could make up.

I wasn't happy inside, watching everyone else be who they wanted to be.
They were all having fun, when inside I was torn apart.

I was headed to some very dark places, but I still couldn't bring myself to tell anyone.
I was afraid of rejection.
I was scared, and very hurt inside.

I didn't realize was that my family was starting to fall apart.

They had less and less family picnics or events, because no one was happy when we were together.

No one knew the reason that I was always so moody, and those special occasions, well, they weren't that special anymore.

They just weren't fun.

They became less and less frequent.

More years went by and I still had all of those same feelings, but each year those feelings got a lot harder for me to deal with. I felt that I couldn't even tell my best friend that I wanted to be a female lion.

I still thought my Mother was beautiful the way she stood proud, like she knew who she was, and was accepted by everyone.

I noticed that other lionesses stood the same, tall and proud with confidence.

All the things of which I was lacking.

I would try to mimic the lioness posture, but I still felt like I was missing something.

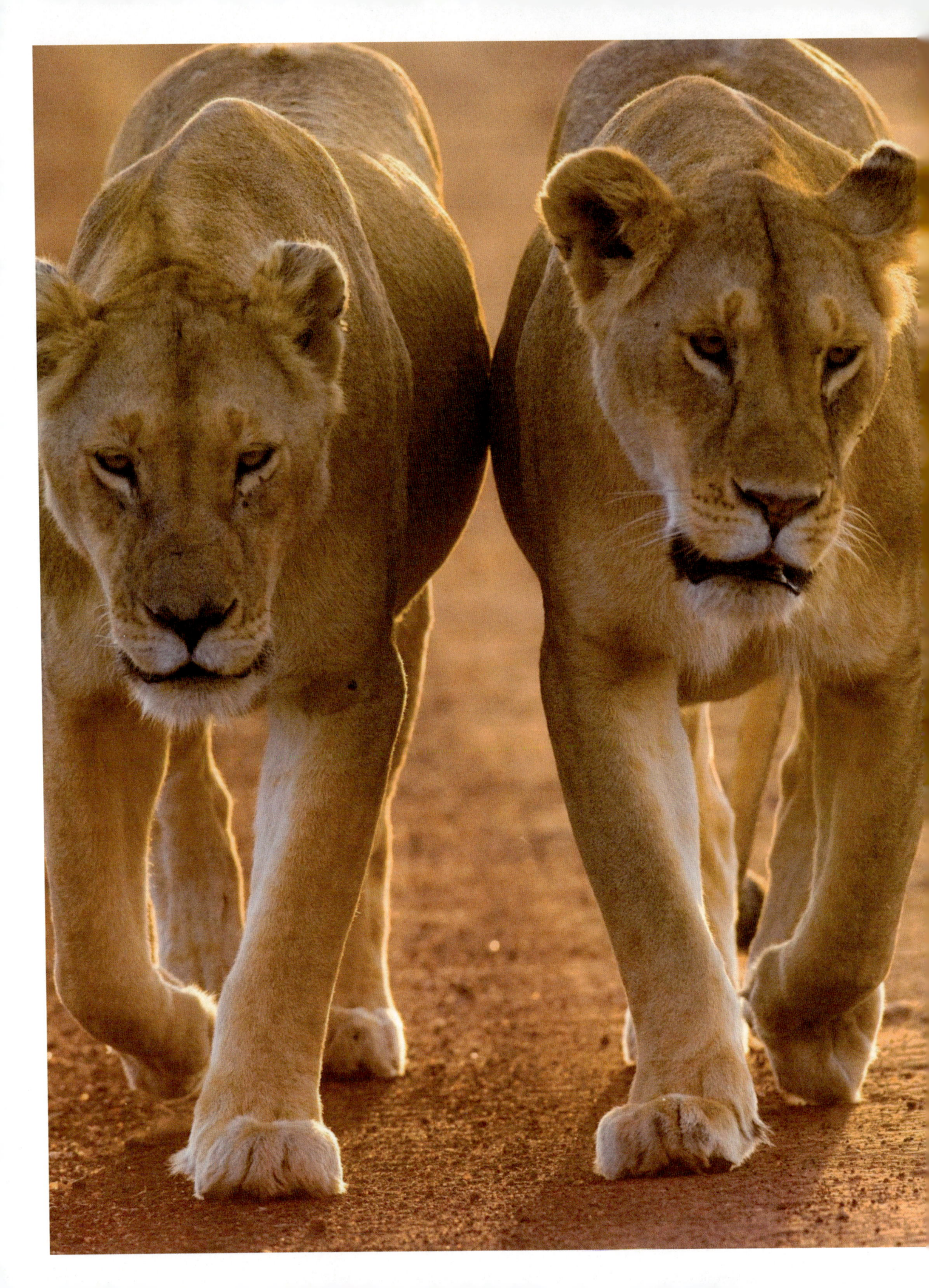

They were magnificent! With all their inner beauty and the way they carried themselves!

The lionesses were so proud of their families, and always had lots of friends.

They felt good about themselves inside and out.

You could tell by their appearances they were whole in both body and mind.

One complete animal, with great vision ahead of them.

I realized what I was missing was a complete body. A body that lined up with my inner self. I had a male lion's body on the outside, with all the emotions and feelings of a lioness on the inside.

I told myself as a lioness I could be all those things.

All of the lionesses were strong inside and proud of who they were.
They didn't have to run around roaring loud, to be noticed or even to be heard.

They were just themselves.

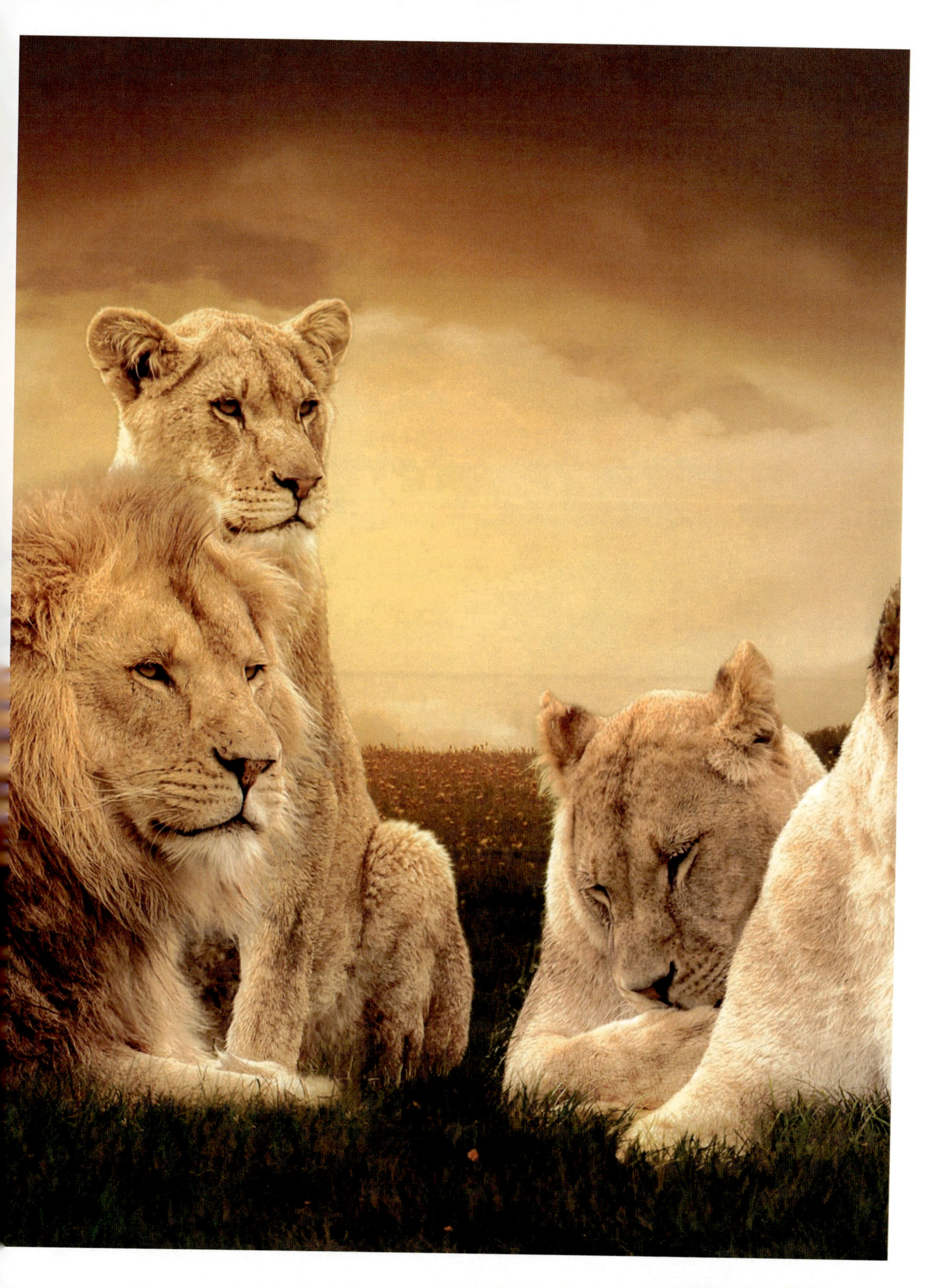

I had started to tell myself that those big fluffy feet were going to be hard to fill.
I was feeling less and less like that was going to be possible.
I was so confused inside!
I just didn't want to live any more!
Why do I have to live like this?
A lioness in a lion's body! The body of a strong brave lion. A lion that was supposed to be King of the Jungle with a roar that everyone would hear, and listen to.
That was just not me! I continued to be alone more and more, cried, and cried more often.
I hated being me!
I hated feeling alone!

I never realized that my Mother had been noticing my behavior and my moods more than anyone else.

For a long time my Mother kept her feelings secret. She knew I was suffering, but didn't know why.

I didn't realize it was tearing her apart too!

She saw the way that I was trying to walk, like a lioness, roar like a lioness, and trying to wear my mane like a lioness.

I wanted desperately to be myself, a female lion, but couldn't get up the courage to tell her, because I was so afraid of losing her, and my family.

I even tried to run away. I had terrible thoughts in my head.

Maybe I shouldn't have been born at all, or maybe I was just born into the wrong family.

Why did I feel this way?

Did they do something to make me feel this way?

NO they did not!

I was born this way!

I would question myself all the time.

I was so unhappy.

Often I would just hide and be by myself. I didn't realize this was the worst thing to do because I would get even more depressed.

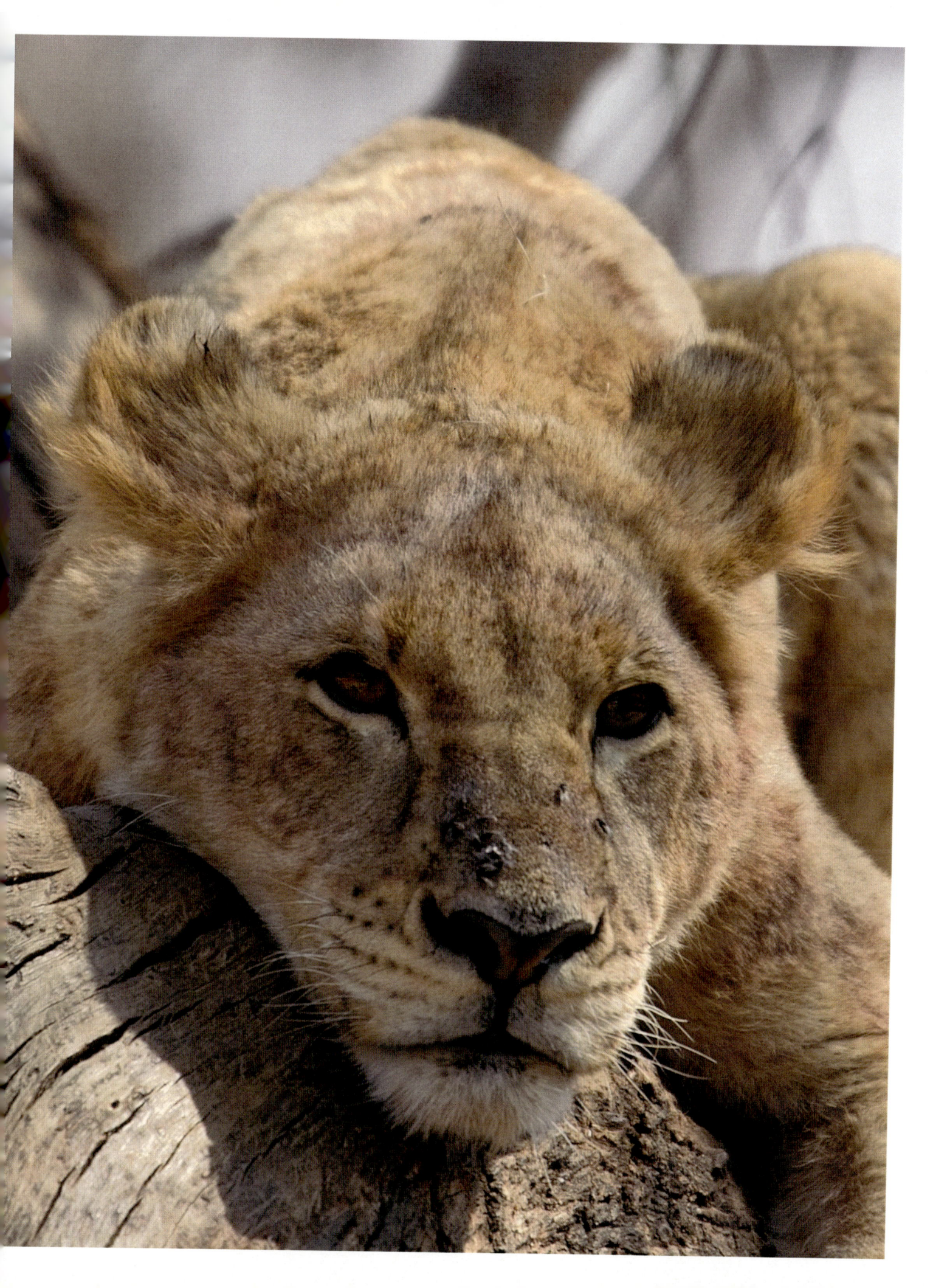

One day my Mother saw me wearing my mane like the other lionesses and said,

"Dillion don't be doing that, everyone will think there is something wrong with you. If you keep doing all of those things that females do, you will lose all of your friends, and the other lions will pick on you.

That is just not how male lions behave! No one will understand, no one!

Your Father and brother and I will be devastated if you keep this up!

This is not funny."

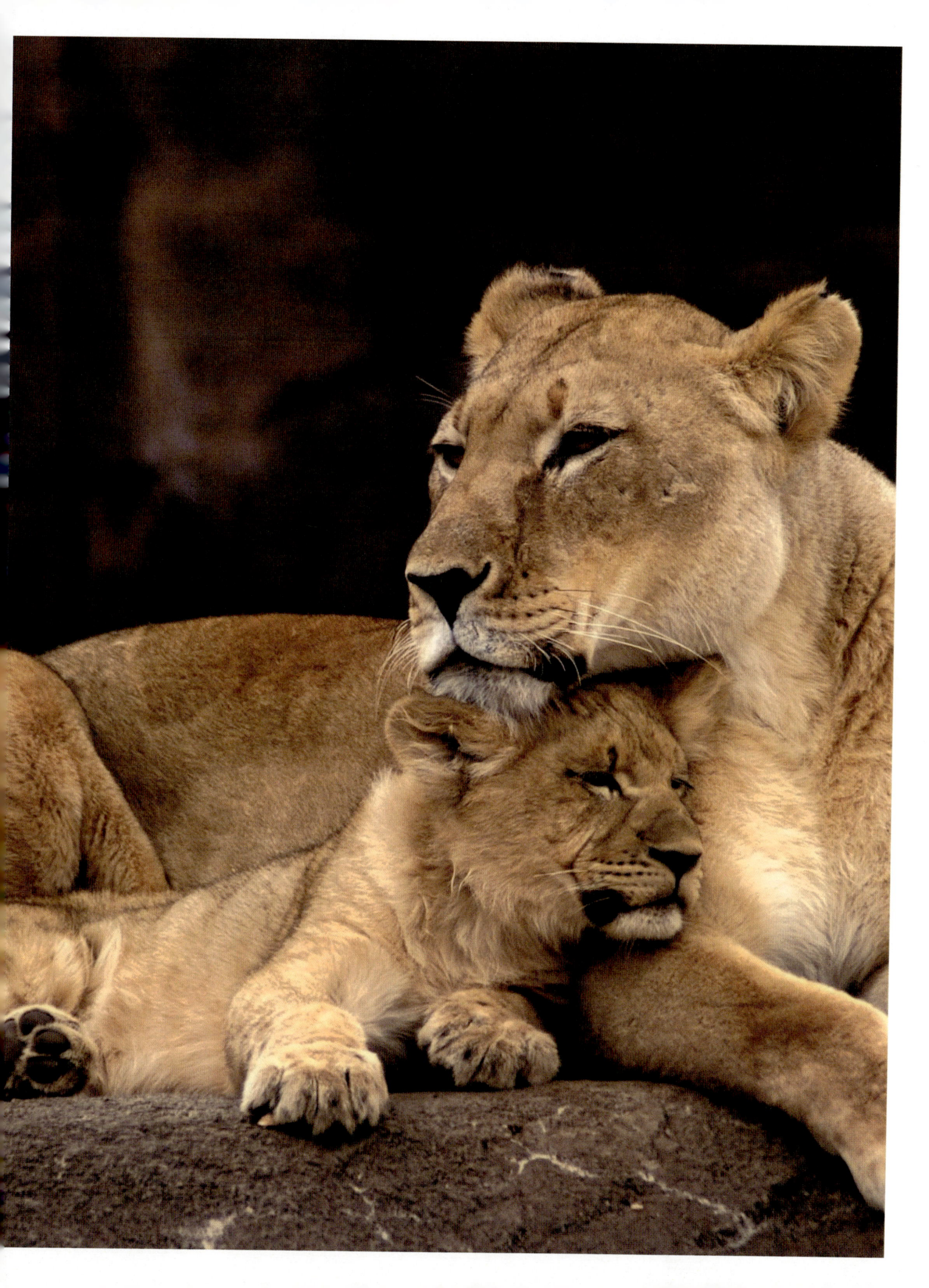

My heart broke even more, when she said those words. I cried inside for a long time.

I thought to myself, I want to look like her, but if I ever have cubs, I won't treat my cubs that way, or say those things.

Can't she see how broken I am?

I am hurting inside, and no one knows why. Are they all blind, and not able to see the real me?

Sometimes I went by myself to a place no other lions would be. I would roar these words out loud.

"I am in here and I just want out! Please help!" I would roar these words out, but I still couldn't say them to anyone else.

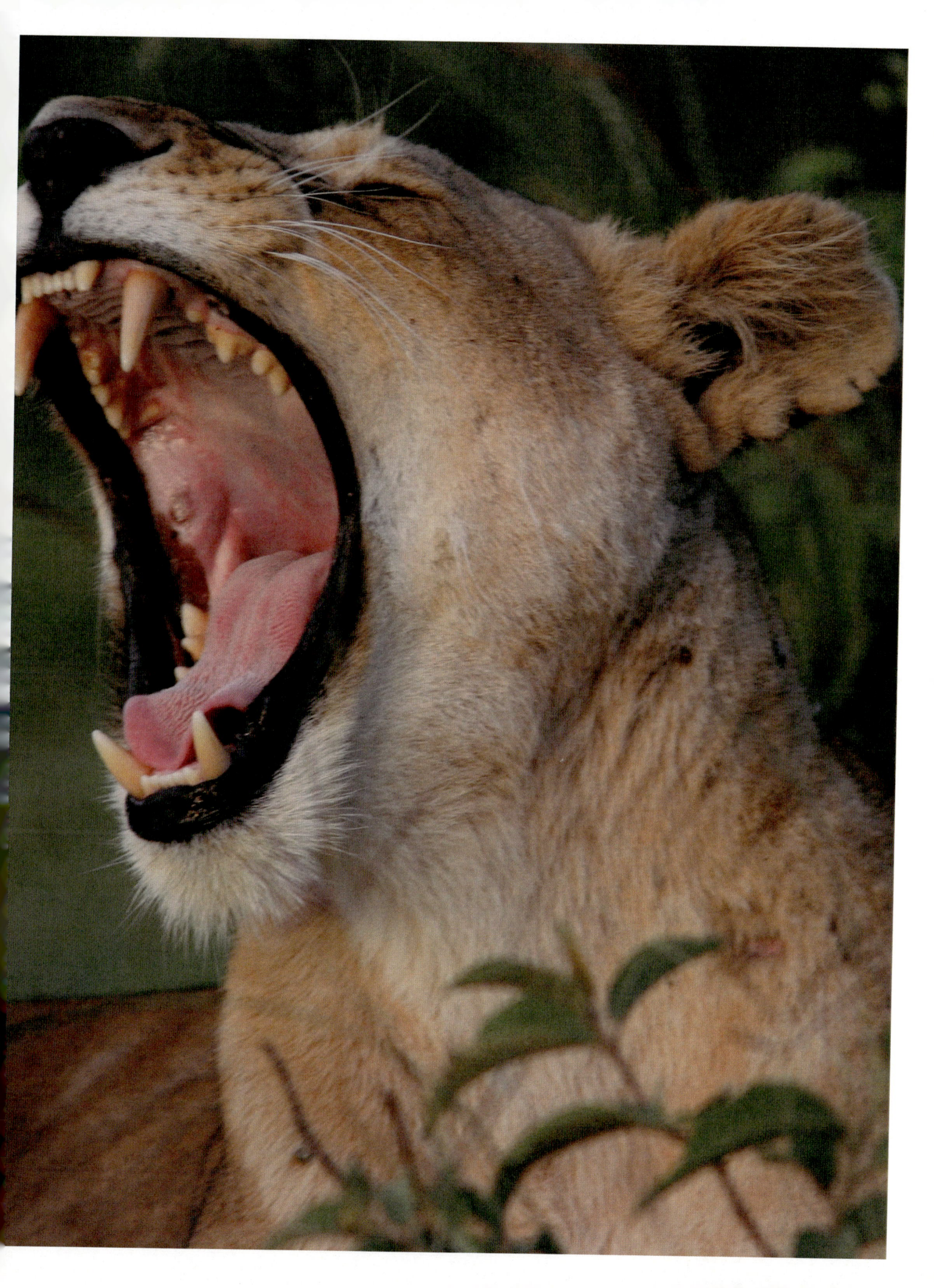

I continued to try to look and act like a lioness, and my Mother would get so mad at me, but I couldn't help it and I couldn't stop myself.

I continued because:

I didn't want to stop!

I wanted someone to find out that I wanted so desperately to be a lioness.

I thought if someone found out it would be easier, that they could tell the world my secret. I thought maybe this would be the easiest way for everyone to find out.

I would ask myself, if someone else told the world about me wanting to be a lioness, would that be the right thing to do?

They would probably all laugh, and bully and harass me, and my family. They wouldn't understand or be able to explain the way I felt.

So hiding and crying all of the time seemed to be what I was best at. "Why do I have to be here at all? Why me?" Again I would ask myself over and over, until I was just making myself sick and weak as a lion, male or female. I was fading inside.

I wanted desperately to be a female lion, not a male lion.

The only part of me that was a male was my body, and I thought that was ugly. I hated the way I looked, and the way I felt.

I wasn't aware of it, but my whole family now knew something was wrong.

Just what, they would have never guessed!

They all thought, or hoped that I would just grow out of that phase in my life. Not one of them realized how badly I wanted to be a female.

Maybe they thought that I was gay, and just wanted a partner of the same sex.

Even that choice, would have been much easier for the lions to accept.

Some of the other lions had chosen partners of the same sex. Although they also had a hard time coming out and telling the world, it seemed to be more acceptable.
My problem was much worse.
At least to me, it seemed that way.
My problem was much different.

My problem was I wanted to transition from a strong masculine male body, to a feminine lioness.
I wanted a different shape and posture, a different sounding voice a different face and beautiful hair.

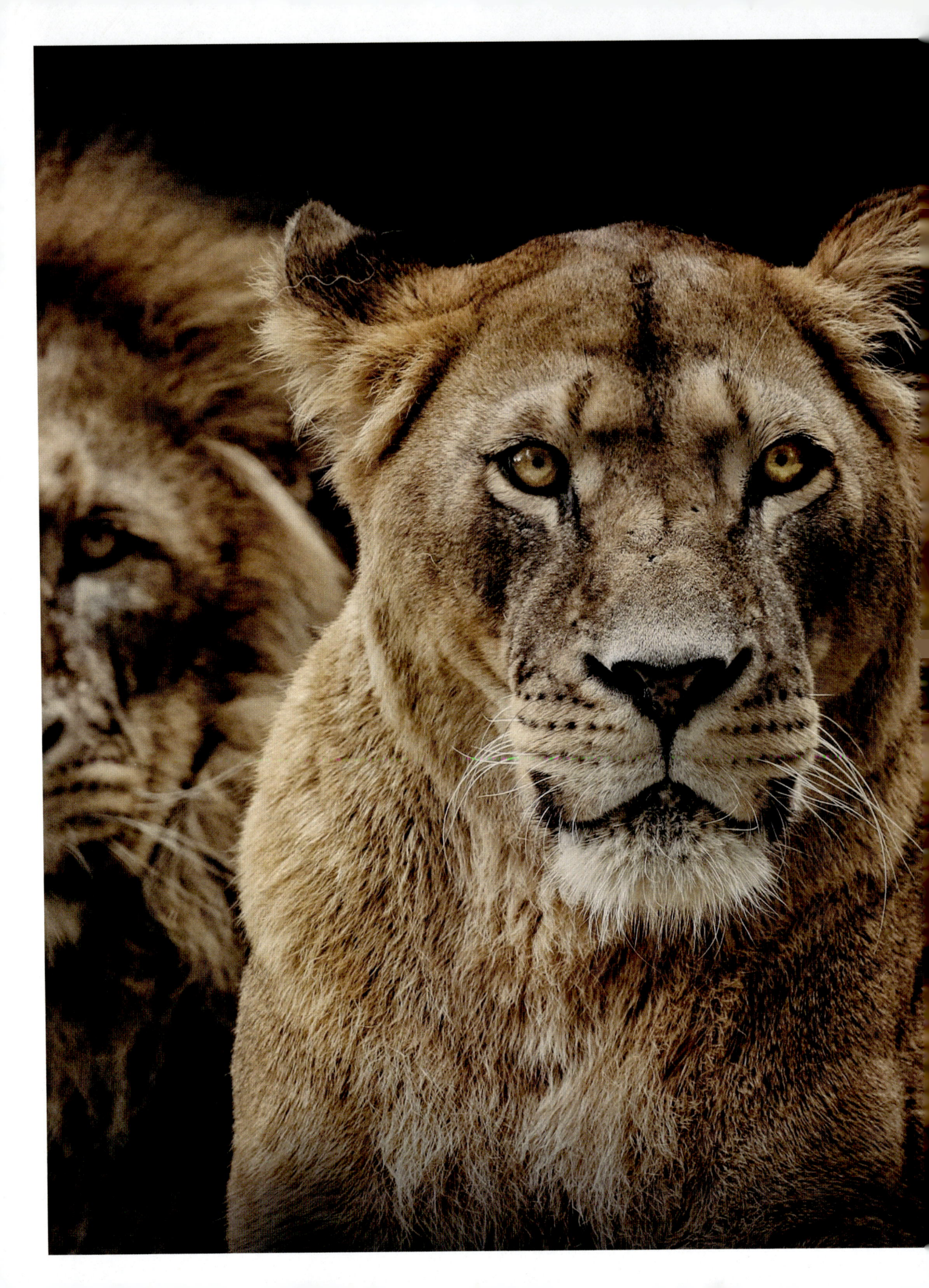

I wanted to change to be the lioness I felt like inside, but I wasn't sure the pride that I was part of was ready to accept that.
So I just continued to fantasize about being a lioness.
I had no doubts!
I was born into the wrong body!

I had a lioness's brain, and a male lion's body, and it was tearing me apart slowly.
I didn't want to be strong and muscular or look handsome.

I didn't care if anyone noticed me or not.

I just wanted to be me!

I wanted to walk like a lioness, and look like a lioness, and let my true female feelings come out.

I wanted to be free! It was tearing me apart inside and out.

I felt broken and ugly and rejected.

I was dying inside, bit by bit. I hated myself, and hated how I looked, but most of all I hated the way I felt.

All I wanted was to be me, a lioness! It was what I wanted more than anything in the world!

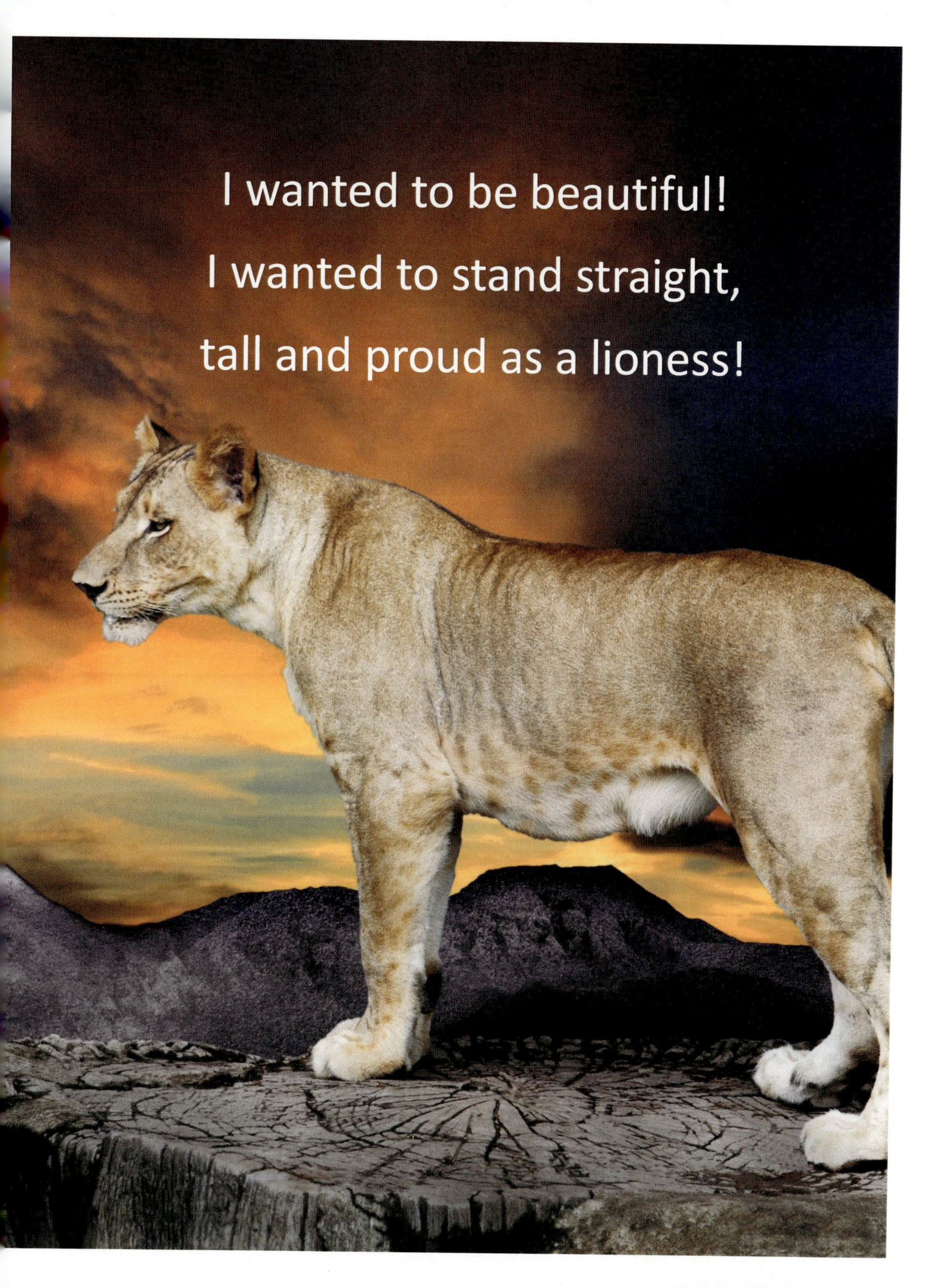

I wanted to be beautiful!
I wanted to stand straight,
tall and proud as a lioness!

I was becoming more and more depressed inside. I no longer liked the way I looked or felt. I still couldn't tell my family or friends.

So most of the time, I would just wander off, to find something that made me feel good, like walking through the wild flowers, and watching birds. Lots of the time, I would hide in a tree or bush, and watch all of the lionesses having fun.

All standing there beautifully!

That would be so wonderful!

I thought to myself, to be so proud of who you are, and not hide your feelings, that would be my dream come true.

.

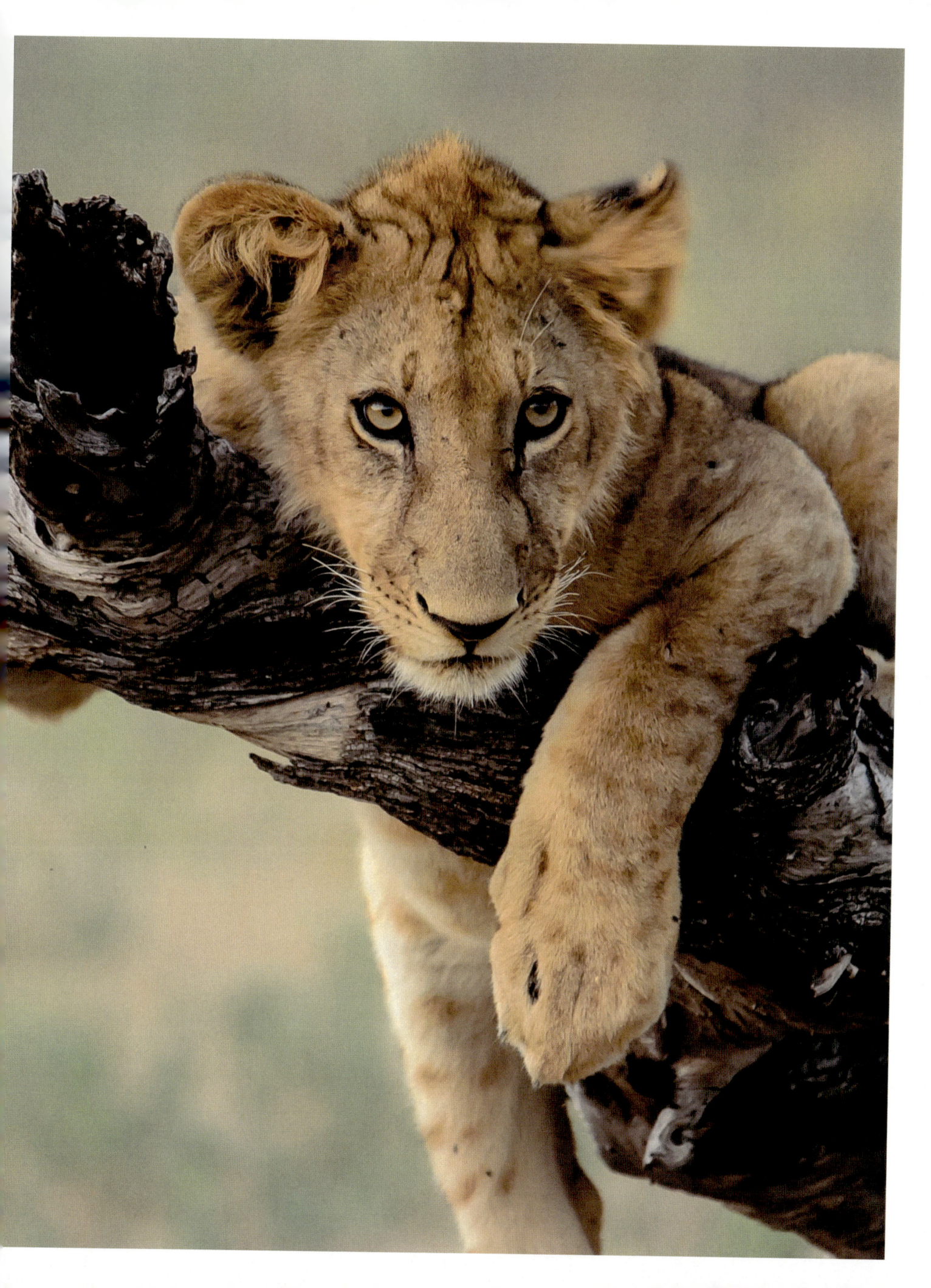

By now I had started to grow my mane, and started to look like a young male lion.

I didn't like this new look at all! Sometimes I would stare at myself in the water pond for a long time telling myself, this is not me! That is not how I see myself on the inside, because I so wanted to be a lioness. Sometimes, I would stare at my reflection. Then get so upset with the way I looked, that I would take my front foot, and stomp in the water! Hoping that when the water cleared that I would see the real me, the lioness I wanted to be, but that never happened. I even wanted to cut my mane off totally, so that I would look like a lioness.

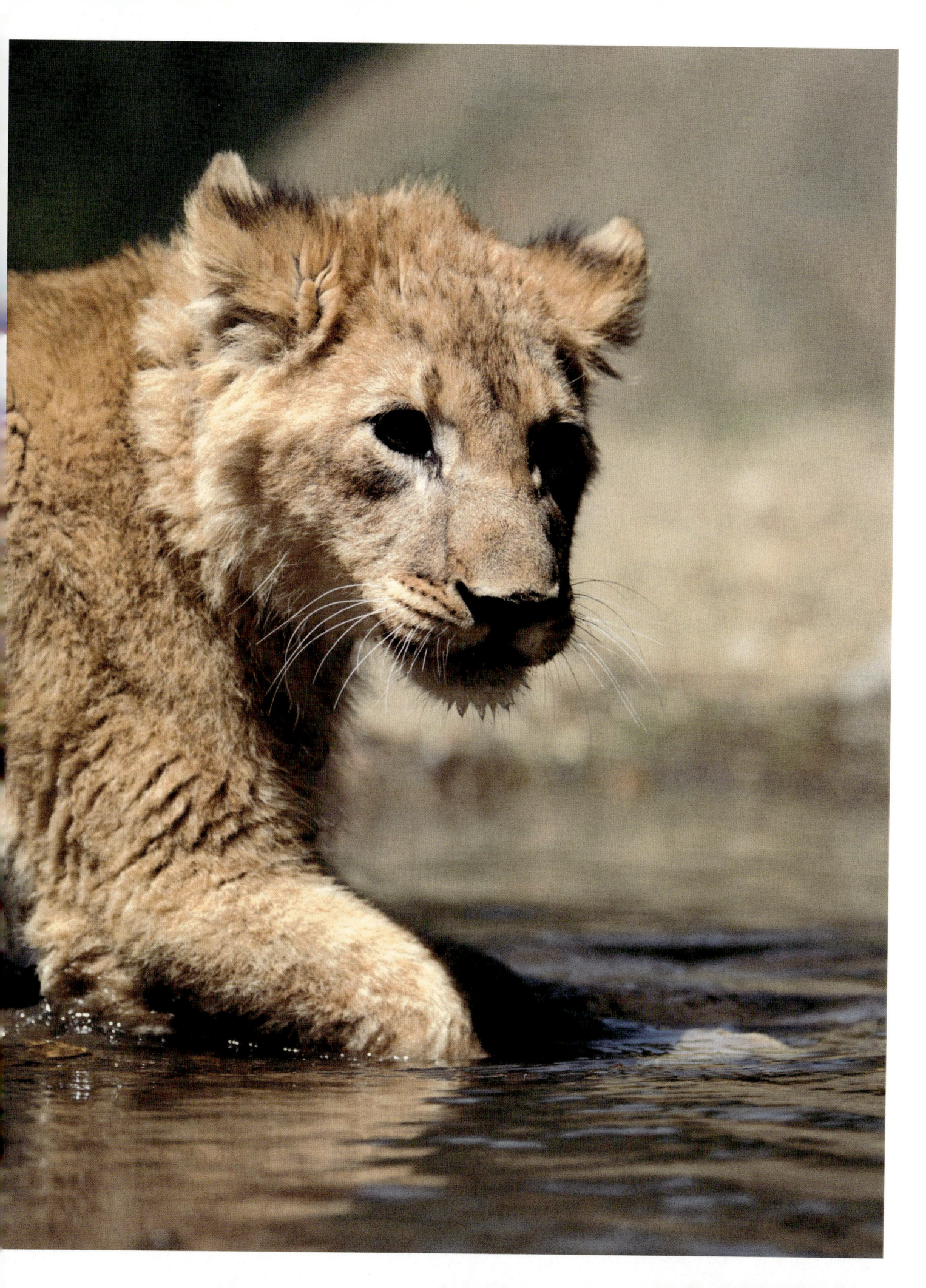

I started to play more and more by myself. Then one day a young female lion came to the waters edge.

I first saw a reflection and thought that it was me!

My wish had come true!

I was now a beautiful lioness!

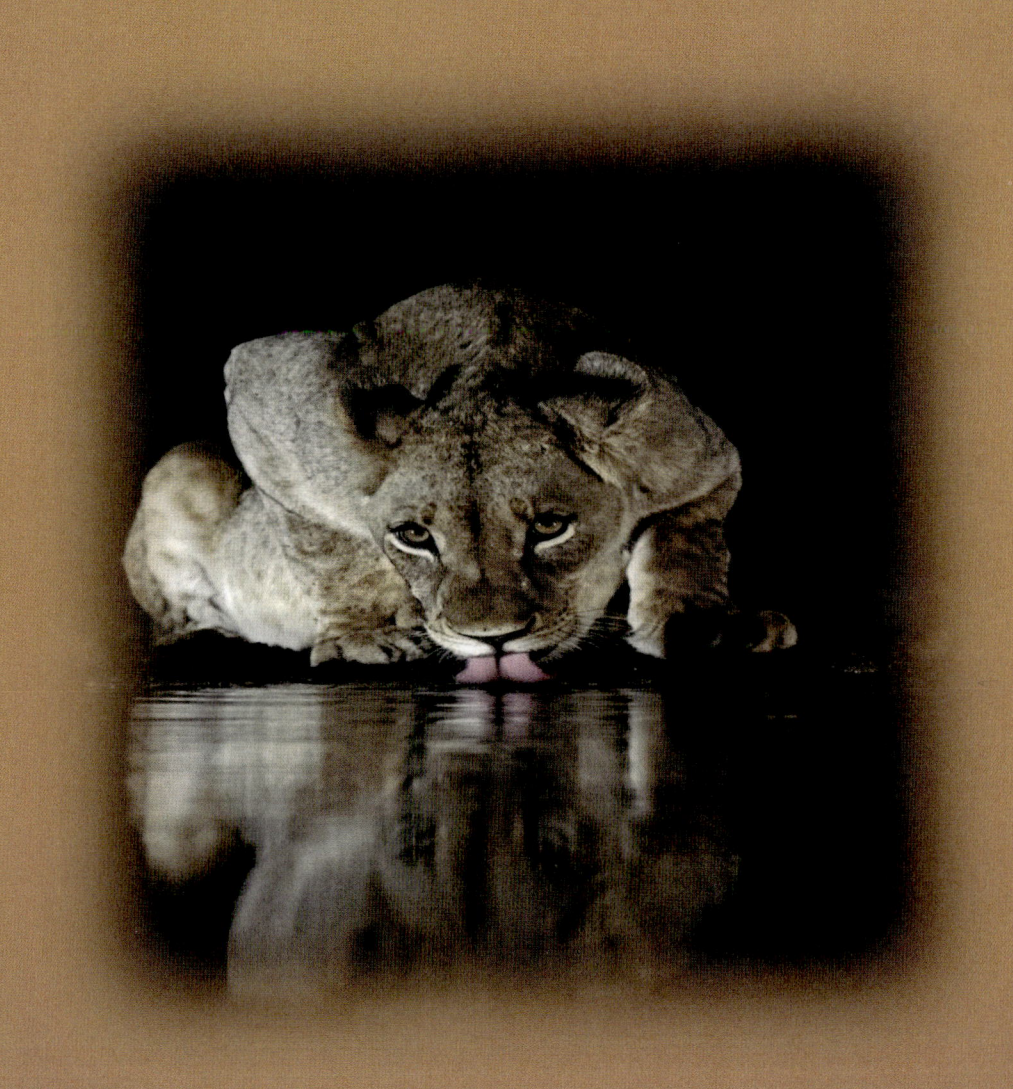

Then the reflection spoke, and I realized it was a reflection of a lioness.

"Hello," she said to me.

"My name is Camilla, who are you?" she asked.

So I answered and told her my name.

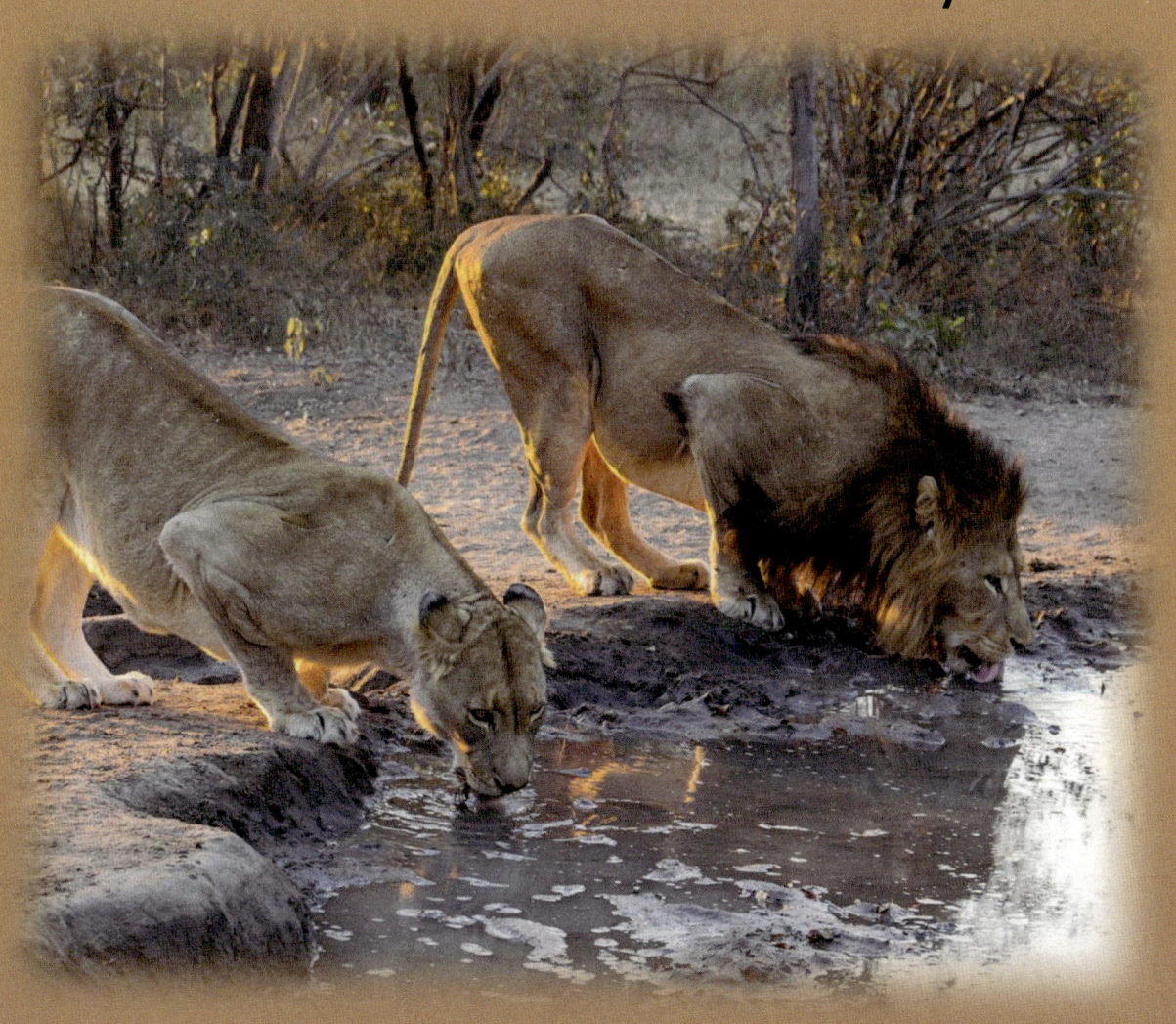

Camilla said, "You are the most handsome lion I have ever seen. Where have you been hiding?" she asked.

I thought to myself, did she know why I was hiding? I had never told anyone!

So I answered, "Oh I have just been around!"

"I just like being by myself a lot."

I replied. " I really don't like lots of lions around me, it makes me feel uncomfortable."

Camilla replied "Me too, I am kind of shy also."

Camilla and I became good friends. We played together, we chased each other around, we hunted together. Sometime, we just roared at each other to see who could roar the longest, and the loudest.

I would always let her win.

It was fun doing all those things!

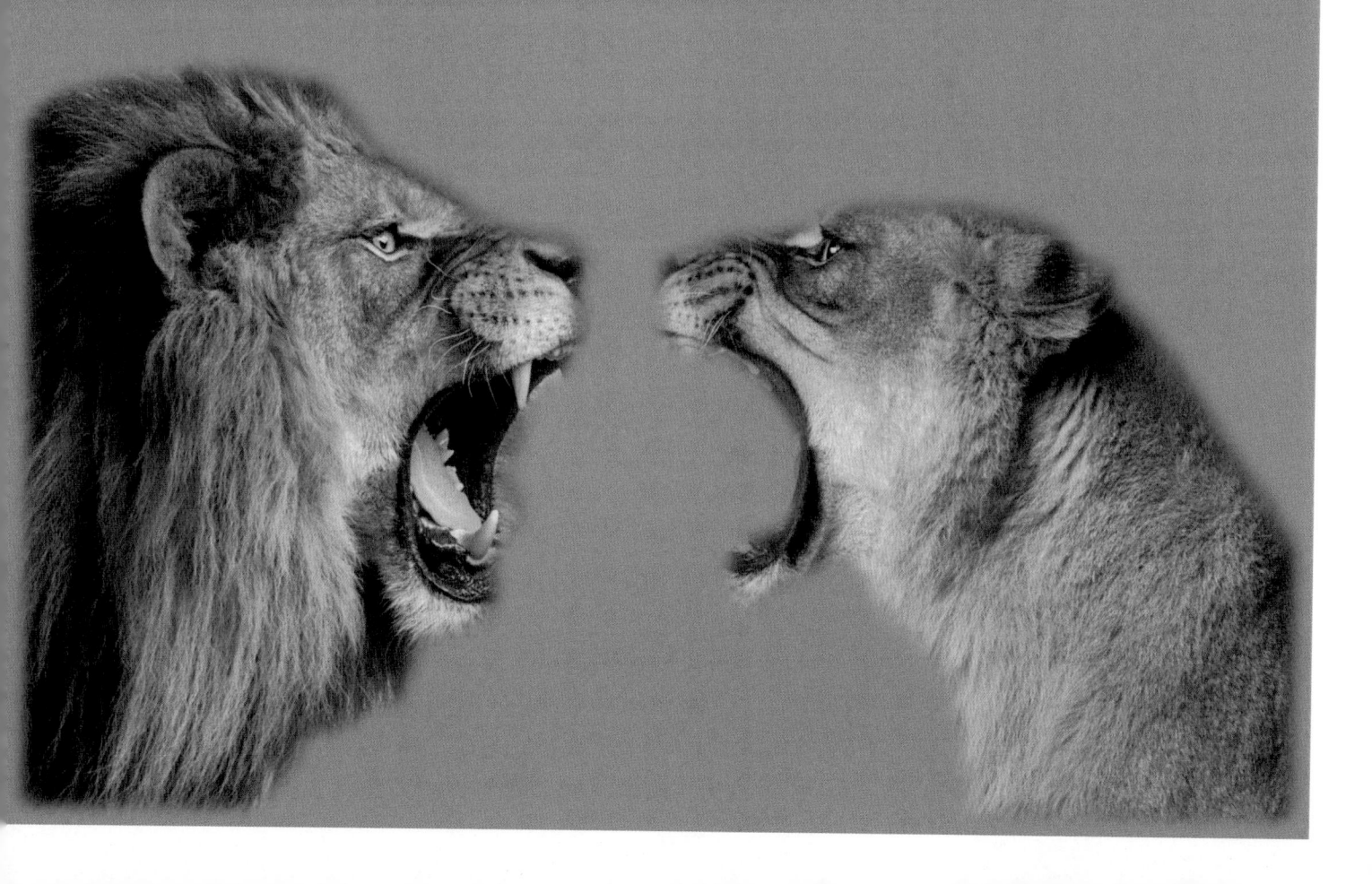

All of the things that female lions do, all the things that I always wanted to do, with the other female lions.

All the things that I was not able to do, and now I was doing them with my best friend, a lioness.

I was finally starting to feel happy, or so I thought.

We made a beautiful couple.

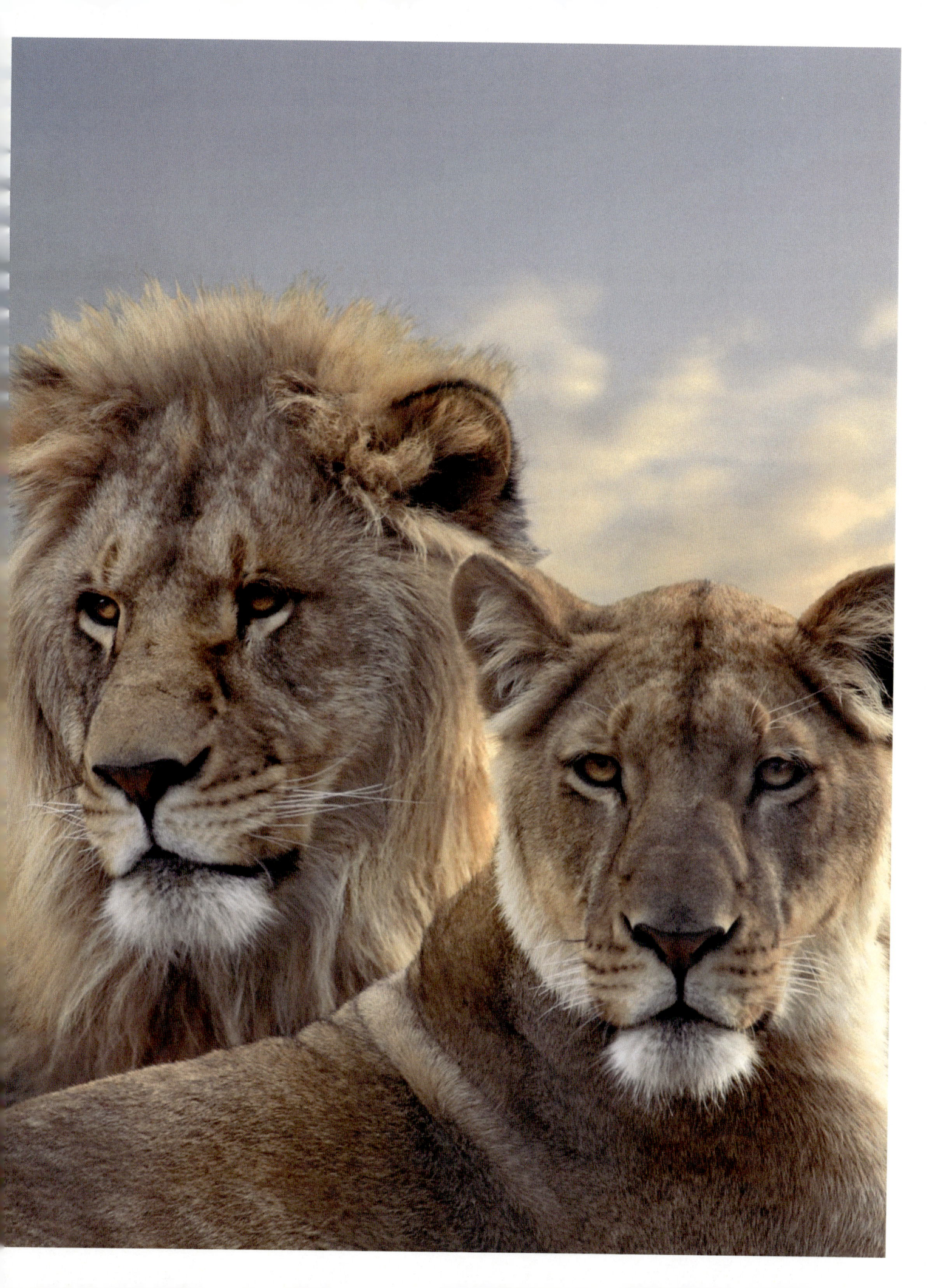

Of course, Camilla never knew how I really felt inside, and I wasn't sure if I could ever tell her. I was afraid of losing her! We had lots of fun together, and now all of those feelings that I had, seemed to disappear.

I told myself: I am no different than the other young male lions,

I just had to mature!

Camilla and I became such great friends, that we became a pair.

Not only did we become a pair. We now had both grown up, and had two young cubs of our own.

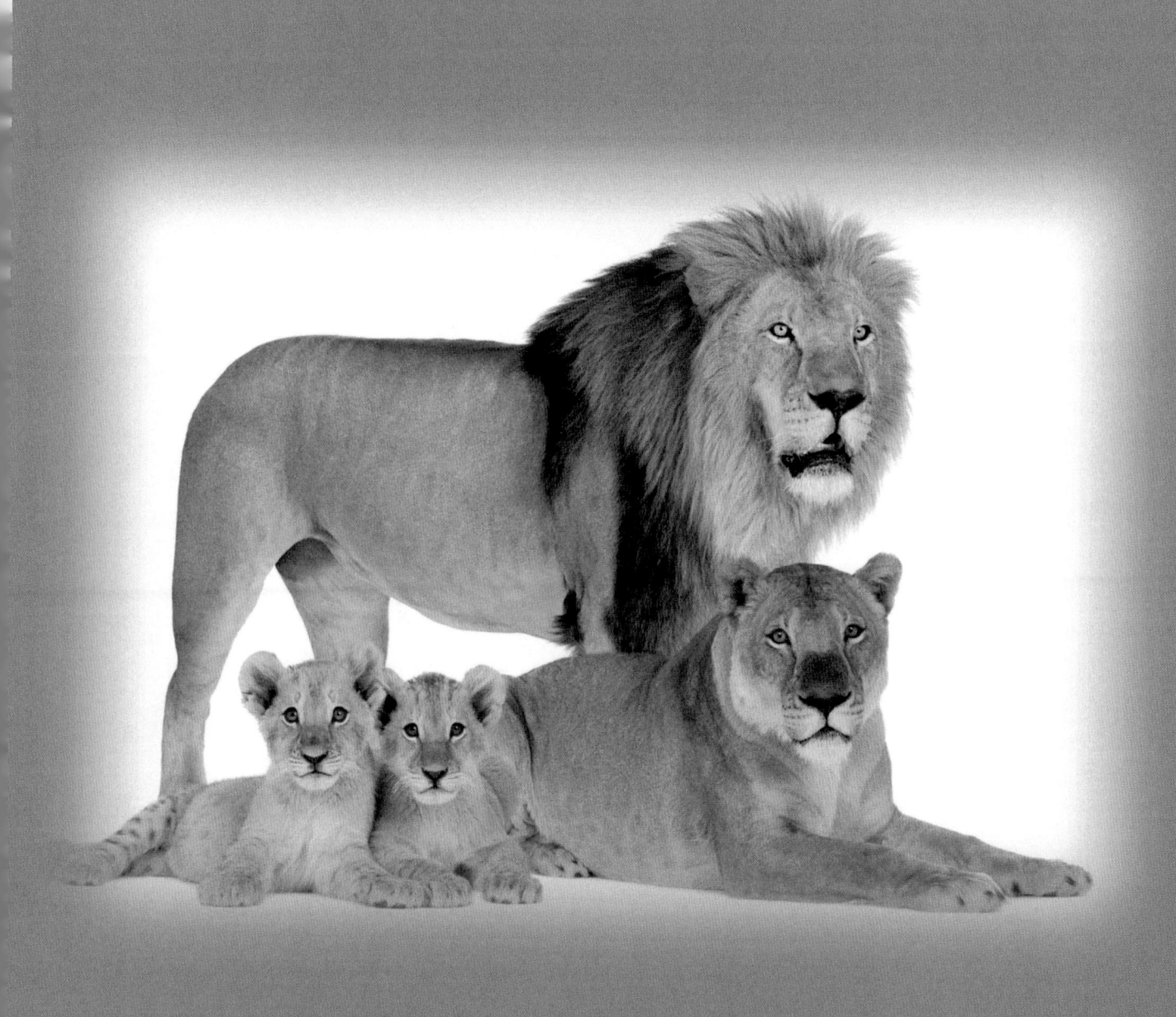

They were handsome.

Two sons, both wrestling with each other, playing and running around.

I loved it!

Inside I felt like a female lion with her baby cubs beside her.

It made me remember when I was that young, doing the same thing with my Mother, my brother, and my Father.

What a wonderful life we had together!

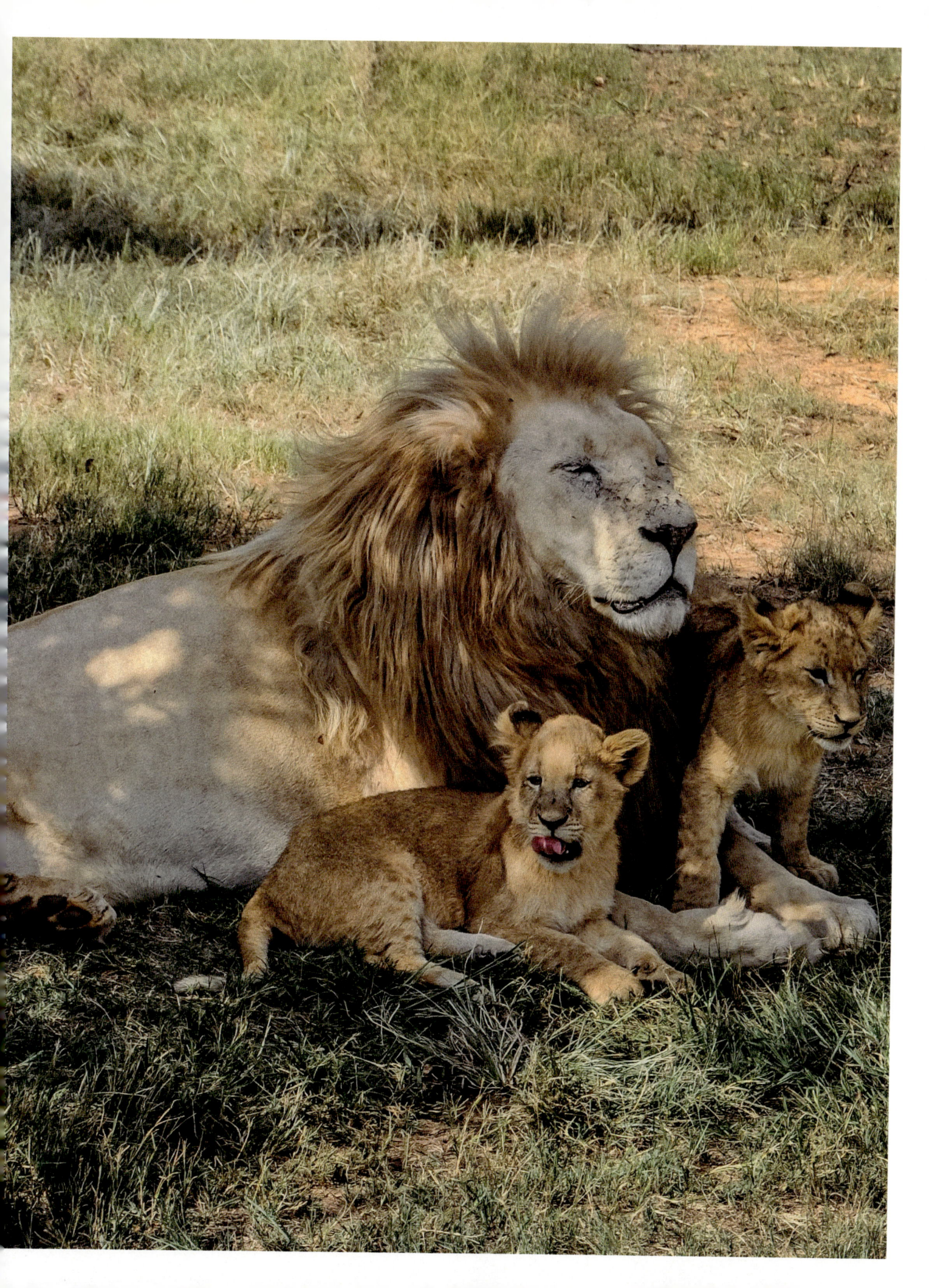

My best friend Camilla, and I parted ways.

I stayed without a partner, and decided that raising my cubs was the most important thing in my life.

I am a great Father, and a very good provider to my sons.

I will always be there for them.

They are number one in my life!

I do everything I can, to prepare them for their future, and to make sure that they are happy today, and will be happy inside and out, tomorrow.

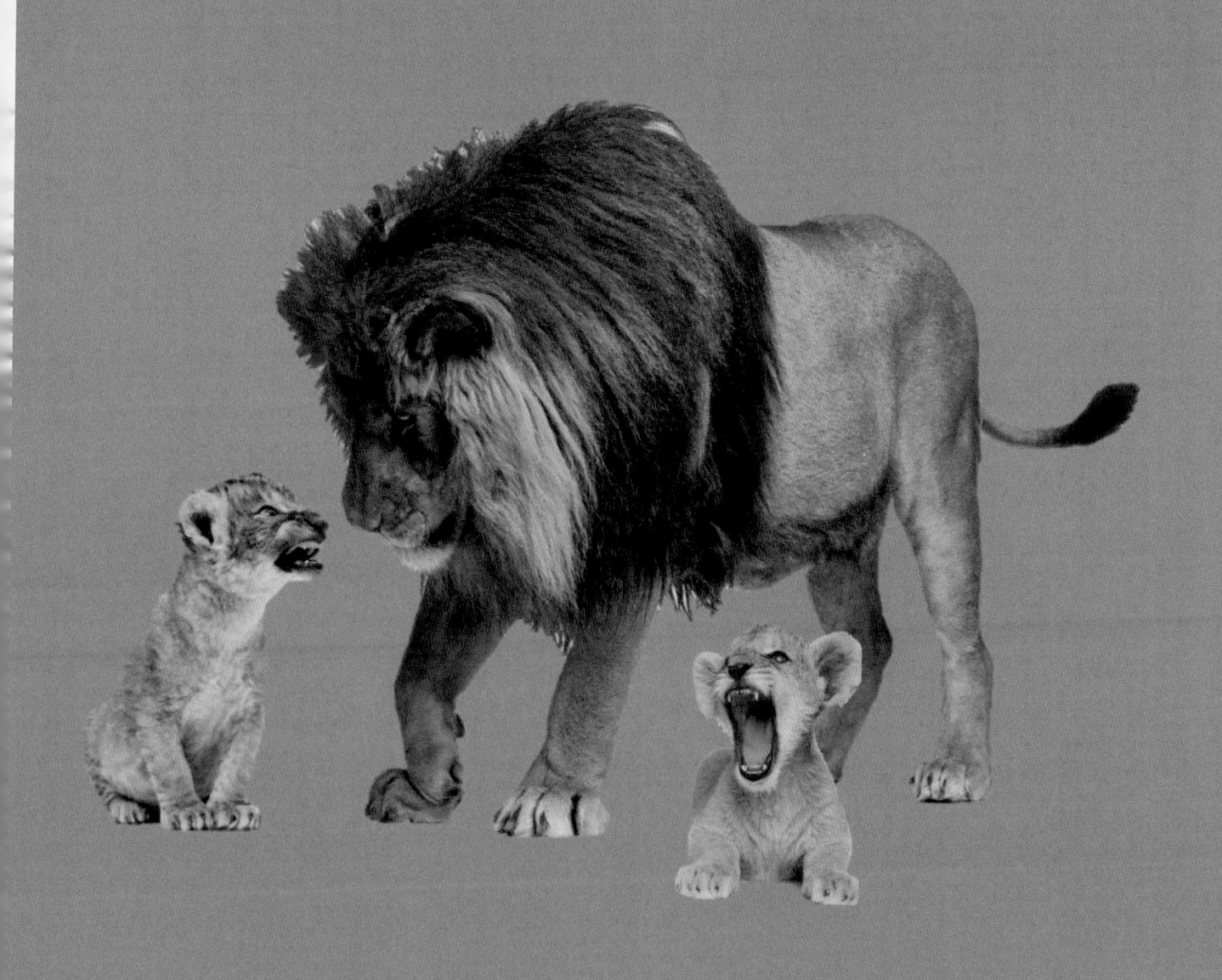

As a Father lion, I knew I had to provide for my family. That meant hunting and doing all of those male things that I never really wanted to do, but now as a single parent I had to do.

I did however, learn that my family comes first.

I needed to take care of my cubs.

They are my responsibility, and my family.

My life is not just about me anymore, it is about my family.

Just as my parents provided for me, I am providing for my cubs.

But deep inside, I still had the same feelings. I never grew out of them, or got over them.

I still felt that I was born into the wrong body.

I had the body of a male lion, but in my heart and my mind, I felt like every other lioness and I still wanted that.

I still hid my feelings, but because now I had my own home with my own cubs, I could let my feelings out more.

I still hadn't told my Mother, or my Father.

I still have those same feelings about being born into the wrong body, but they are stronger than before.

I have not yet figured out a way of telling the world, that I don't want to be alone any longer!

I don't want someone coming and taking my two cubs away, because of who I am or how I feel inside.

So again, I still continued to hide my feelings for a few more years.

My two cubs have grown up now. They are nine and ten. I speak with honesty, but yet with dignity, when I talk to my sons, because I do not want my sons to be judgemental of others.

So, we have many discussions about my changes. They have the right to know, before anyone else does.

I love them both dearly!

We know other male lions, that have chosen to have other male lions as their companions, and other female lions, whom have chosen other female lions to be their companions also. Some of them have cubs of there own or have adopted cubs. They are all wonderful lions and lionesses and live very happy lives.

Those lions and lionesses will not make fun of me. They understand just how it feels to be different, and the need to be yourself.

All I want is to be me! Happy, loving, caring, and a great parent to my cubs.

There will be lots of other male and female lions that will never understand how I feel. It is very hard to try to explain my inner feelings to anyone, because most lions male, or female don't want to listen.

I understand that they may not accept me, although I am still me! I feared they might not even let my cubs play with theirs, or they may harass the ones I love the most.

There is a lot to think about, but what I know is that many nights,

I still cry myself to sleep!

I just want to let the loudest roar out to the world:

"Look deeper inside, please just look at me, and let me come out!

I am female and I am very proud of it! I really don't care how you see me, for I see myself so differently than you do!

I am very hurt, and crying inside.

I cry everyday, and have for many years!

I am afraid that everyone I love will leave me, because they can't accept me for who I am not what I am!"

There is nothing to be afraid of,

I am still me!

I want to change the way I look, to the way I feel inside, and that is from a lion to a lioness.

Other lions will definitely notice the change, and may not like it.

I cannot live like this any longer.

I either end my life today, or Roar!

So today is the day!

I decided that I could not continue to live like this any longer!

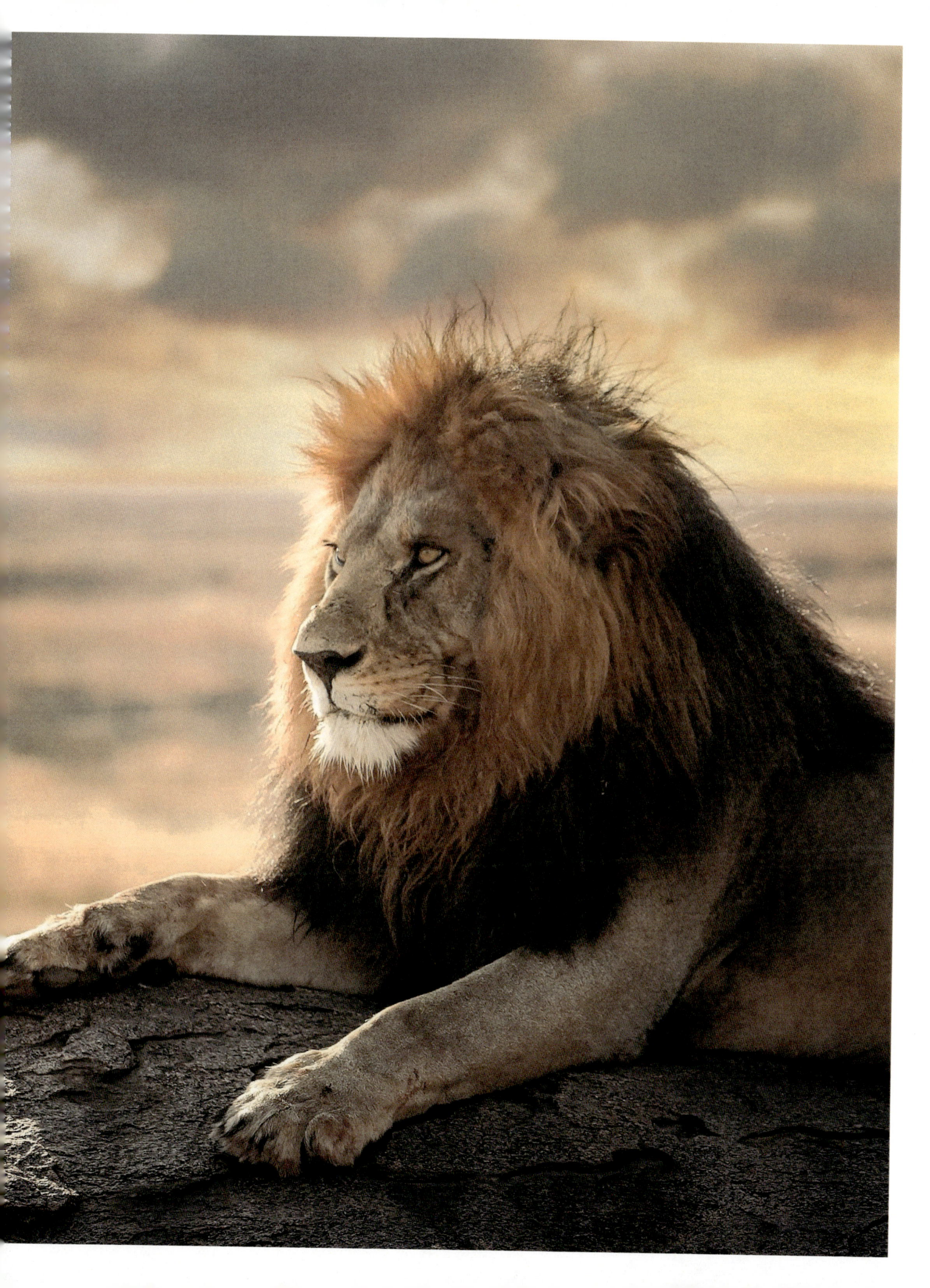

My Name is EDREI!

meaning

Strong and Powerful.

I want to live! I want to be happy, and live a healthy life. I need to take care of my cubs, and myself!

So today!

I am ready to ROAR!

I am coming out, like it or not!

I will not be a broken lion inside

or out anymore!

I eat the same as you,

I think the same as you,

I provide for my family like you.

I love my cubs, the same as you!

I am still the same lion,

I will just have a new look.

I am not asking you to make a fuss over me, or try to go out of your way to please me. I am still the same lion!

I just have a fresh new look, and that fresh new look will make me a much happier lioness inside and out!

I am proud to be part of pride, and

I will stand up, and stand alone

if I have too!

I do this not for you.

not for my friends,

but for myself!

I am me, I am EDREI!

strong and powerful!

So bring on the world, and

more lions like me!

Lets make the loudest ROAR

you have ever heard.

Let the world hear us because

we stand together, as a group called

PRIDE!

I have since told my Mother and my Father, and my brother.
I was unsure as to what their reaction would be. I didn't think I could face them because of the hurt I thought I was putting them through.
I expected rejection, laughter, remarks, and humiliation.
I didn't want to hurt them because I love them, with all my heart, whichever body, my heart was in.

It was still my heart, and my soul.
I love them all, my parents, my brother, my sister-in law, my children and my extended family and friends!

I received unconditional love, support and understanding.

I can't express just how much that means to me.

I just can't find the right words.

Now I cry, tears of joy,

I cry because

I am so proud of them!

because they did not reject me, and letting me slip away.

I love them all!

Words, just aren't enough!

You don't have to be the biggest,

or the bravest

King of the Jungle

to make the

loudest Roar!

You just have to be the

Proudest Lion,

in the Pride,

to make an Impact!

I am sure it was a shock to them, as they all knew that I liked acting like a lioness.

No they weren't happy with me doing that!

Yes, there was a lot of very hurtful conversations between us over the years.

Them not understanding me, and me not understanding them.

I always thought that I would be a disappointment to them.

I have apologized over and over again, for doing so.

Their response was, "You are not, nor have you ever been a disappointment to us.

It is just disappointing to us, that you have held all of those feelings inside for so many years, and suffered so badly, and that you thought you were a broken lion, and that we misunderstood each other."

My Mother said, "We were very lucky to have two cubs born into this world, and we will always have two cubs. Regardless of their sex, or choice of partner they choose in their lives."

I have told them that I had started the transition. I just couldn't live like that, duel male/female thing anymore.

It was tearing me apart, and I know that I have many happy long years ahead of me, with my two cubs.

Also, with lots of lions and lioness in my my life that love me, just for me!

I know that I will lose some of my friends, best friends, and family members, but I also know that along the way, I will make new friends.

Friends, and family members that will stand behind me throughout my journey.

I know that my two sons are going to find it hard to face at first, but they are me, they are part of me, and I will always love them, regardless of what they choose in their lives.

They will grow up stronger, knowing that they have a choice to be what they need to be in life.

This is my story!
A true story, and I am hoping that by sharing my story with others, that maybe I could save even just one person, from going to dark places, or doing desperate things to themselves or others, because they were scared or ashamed.

Do not be ashamed of yourself, whomever you are, on the inside.

The only person in your life, that has to be happy to survive, is you!

It was the hardest day of my life when I decided to tell my parents, and my brother.
I couldn't face them to tell them so I sent a letter to them in an email.

The letter below is the email that I sent my family.
I wrote it over and over again, it seemed like one thousand times, to find the right words, but finally I realized it had to come from my heart.
The following letters are all my own words.

I Love You All!

Family.
I know you are thinking, what is this letter! So I'll get right to the point.
For year's I've suffered from anxiety and depression and have been to some really dark places in my life.
You all know I've dressed up in women's clothing before, its not a fad, or influenced by others.

I can't help it: I was born this way!

For years now, I've always thought that I was the only person like this, always struggling with my identity.
Always asking myself, what is wrong with me, why can't I be normal?

There was never a day that went by,
I didn't think about ending my life.
I was always afraid of coming out because of rejection from family, and friends.
I was always told, if I continued dressing up like that:
Don't ask us for help!
You will not get the boys!
We are moving!
People will make fun of you!
You will be an embarrassment to us
And plenty more.
Its tough to be myself, when I'm always given negativity and never asked to sit down and chat.

So last year in Feb. I went to a very dark place, but I thought really hard about it.
I thought about my kids, and my family.
I decided to choose being happy.
I want to see my kids grow old!
So I went to the Doctor and he sent me to the Family Health Team.
I started hormone replacement therapy last May 2018, and have been extremely happy with no bad thoughts anymore.
I know you don't understand it, and we can sit down with the Doctor or the Family Health Team and talk.
I love you guys more then anything, but I need to be happy.

I know it'll take time to adjust to me.
In May I went to Port Elgin for Pride Week, and Pride Conference to learn more about myself, and to meet other trans people and see what issues they had coming out.
A lot of the same kind of stories, suicide, depression and anxiety.
I had a great childhood, and family, but something was always missing.
I always felt different.
I was always feeling lonely.
I am emotionally, and physically drained!
It's always on my mind, how to tell you and what you will think.
You didn't fail as a parent, or a brother, its just who I am, I want to be happy!

Please accept me, for who I am.

I also wrote a coming out letter to my fellow employees.

Letter.

Dear Employer, and Fellow Employees:
Over the last 35 years I've suffered from anxiety, depression and have been to some really dark places in my life.
The reason I'm sharing this with you is because I want to educate you all on what I am going through.
I started (hrt) hormone replacement therapy last May 2018, which means I will be transitioning from male to female.

I will not answer any questions about surgeries. Don't worry about using the wrong pronouns, or name right now.
I won't take offense to it, and if you are unsure, just ask.
The reason for coming out now, was I was heading to a very dark place and I wanted to be happy.
Our Employer, and our Union as well as our LGBT committee, and some friends at work, know about me.
My family knows and supports me 100%.

I feel like I will have a stronger relationship with my family, now that I'm not hiding anything.

For years I've always felt different, like I don't fit in, with any type of group. I know a lot of people will be wondering, why I hid it for so long. Why, have you decided to come out now?
I've always wanted to come out, but was afraid of rejection, maybe losing my family, my kids and my friends. So far, the people I have told have been extremely supportive.
I know I will be the talk of this company for the next 30 years lol, but I am open, and I will try to answer any questions you have about trans issues.

This is the hardest thing I've ever done in my life. I have felt this way since I was 7 years old.

I am doing this for myself, to be happy and to see my kids grow old. My kids have been extremely supportive as well.

This isn't the way I was brought up, or my family's fault, or influenced by others.

I was born this way!

I tried for years to fit in, and be normal. I got married and had kids, but something was missing in my life.

I know that a few of you won't accept me and that's fine, I know its new to our plant.

With me coming out now,
I might just help someone else who is scared.
I would love to be a role model, for others to look up to, so they know I made it safe for them to come out, and not be afraid, and they can be themselves.
Everyone I've told has said, you are so brave for doing this, but I don't see it that way.

I am scared as hell to do this!
But I have to do it, to be happy.
.

I will probably be coming to work in the fall as a female, so if anyone has a problem with me, you can talk to me, our union or our employer.
I will be changing my name to:

Jennifer.

Pronouns, she and her.

I myself have struggle for many years. The youngest memories for me started when I was 7, I am now 44. I always knew that I was female, but if I had told someone, anyone!

I probably would have been label as having a mental disability years ago.

This is not a mental disability.

I struggle from what is known as Gender Dysphoria.

Gender dysphoria is discomfort, unhappiness, or distress due to one's gender or physical sex.

Gender dysphoria is no longer consider to be a mental disorder, but rather the emotional state of distress, which results from the gender identity.

Conditions:

One feels that your body does not reflect your true gender. This can cause severe distress, anxiety and depression. "Dysphoria" is a feeling of dissatisfaction, anxiety, and restlessness. With gender dysphoria, the discomfort with your male or female body can be so intense that it can interfere with your normal life, for instance, at school or work or during social activities.

This also effects other people around you, as they do not understand your state of mind, and a lot of people are unwilling to accept you.

Letters of Support from Friends and Family.

1. Jennifer! It's your cousin in Toronto!
My sister connected with me today and shared your letter, and I'm so excited, and proud that it's hard finding words right now.
There is absolutely no courage without fear, and any fear that you've had or will have can only make your courage stronger.
Look at what you have achieved:
you are showing up to life with a bravery that is incredibly rare.
I look up to you and I'd love to keep chatting at some point!
I send LOVE and PRIDE your way today and always.
I can't wait to see you again sometime and have a proper catch up. I'm off to World Pride tomorrow in NYC and when I march, it will be for you!

2. I admire you Jennifer it takes a very brave courageous person to finally be the person whom you were meant to be! You have my support and I will be here for you whenever you need some one.

3. Wow Jennifer, I support you 100% you were one of the first ppl I met at work, and always treated me as an equal, never talking down to me or making me feel stupid, and I consider you a good friend. You've been there for me when I need to talk, and I can't thank you enough. Your courage is unbelievable! I'm happy for you, that you are out of your dark place, being there is hard and not many understand anxiety and depression. I always felt we would have been labelled.

4. How I have seen you grow in these past few months as you have taken on this courageous journey to FINALLY be your TRUE SELF is an inspiration... Words can not express how proud we are of you... My wife and I are honored to say Jennifer is our friend.

5. Jennifer! An inspiring letter from an inspiring woman. I'm so happy for you. Love and hugs. ♥ ♥ ♥.

6. Very proud of you. You have always been loved and will always be loved no matter what. You are like my own child and I will always be here for you!

7. Jen... You are beautiful... Love ya!

8. Be happy! That's all that matters. I am glad you shared with us. Nothing but support here 👏.

9. I'm so happy, you are finally going to be able to be you. I have felt for years that you were in a bad place, because you couldn't be who you wanted to be. The only way is up now. **Congrats.**

10. Jennifer, I can only imagine the pain and black depression you have lived with and hidden from the world. I hurt for you my friend!
Always with a smile and joke, now I see your defence.
This is a huge step towards healing your heart, and your peace of mind, and I wish you well Jen. Life takes so many twists and turns some good, some bad. Always remember you have a strong support system now, use it!!!
You have shown unbelievable inner strength and I support your new journey and respect your decision Jennifer.
PS: I love your middle name!!!

This list goes on and on, with people all supporting Jennifer, who was loved all this time and didn't know it.
The support groups are many, and the Doctors, and the therapist are excellent.
Family is extremely important at this time, and yes I have shared many a tear with all.
I only have one regret, and that is that Jennifer didn't come home sooner, but the world wasn't ready for this lioness yet.
So here she comes!
I am Woman! Hear me Roar!:
by Helen Reddy,
Is the perfect song choice for both this book and Jennifer Edrei Brown.

Transgender Flag

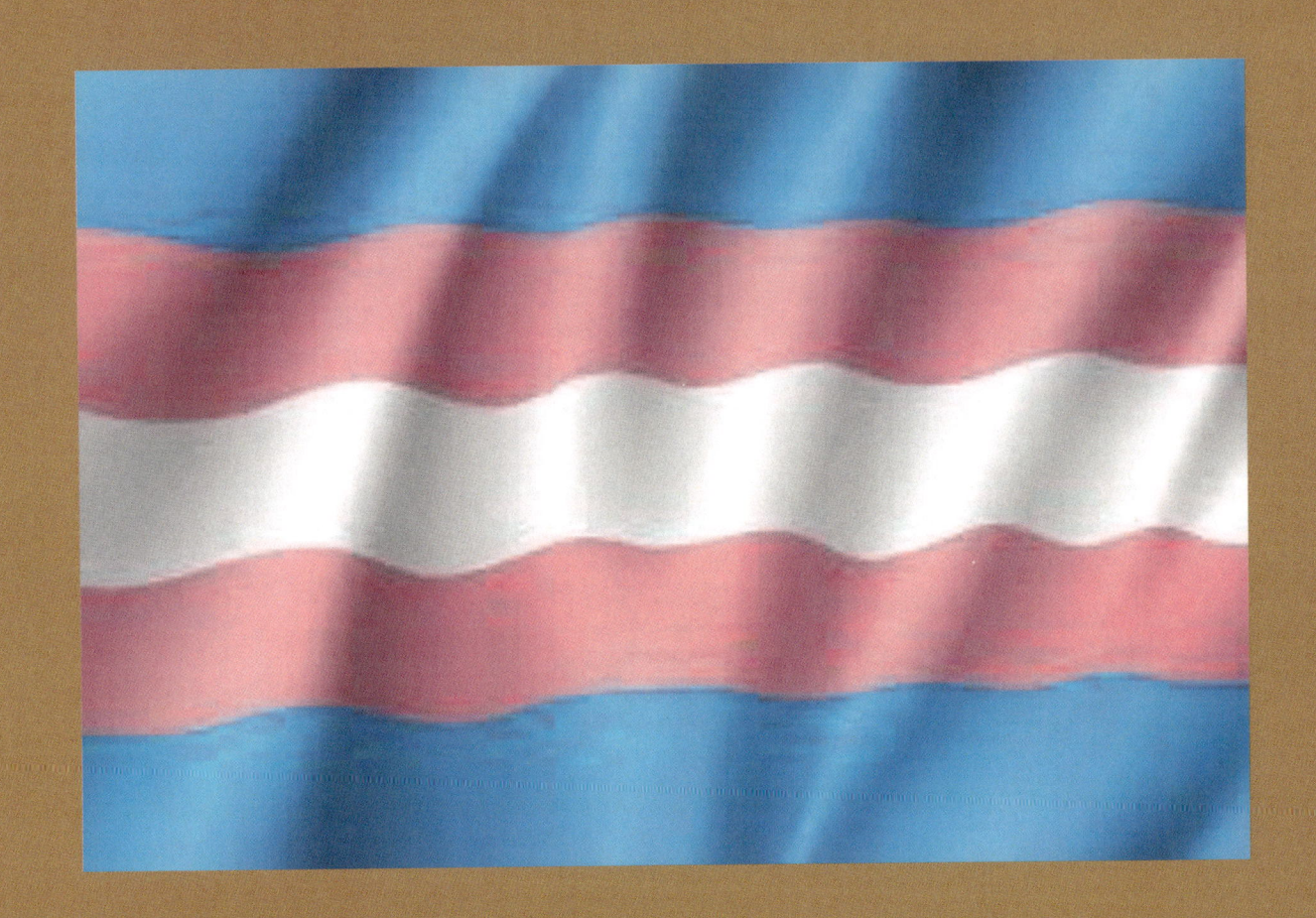

What does LGBTQ stand for? LGBTQ is an acronym for **lesbian, gay, bisexual, transgender and queer** or questioning.

Transitioning:
Is the process of moving from one gender to another. This is known as "transitioning." When a person wants to transition and is able to do so, dramatic improvements are seen in their mental health and work productivity. This is true despite facing "high levels of mistreatment."

Gender dysphoria is not "contagious": sexual orientation and gender identity are not inherited or "passed down" from parents to children. The social stigma around being trans can also be challenging for the family.

The best ways to confront these challenges include learning as much about trans experience as possible to dispel any myths and misconceptions, seeking out support from counselors, and friends and being willing to communicate with care and honesty.

Everyone has the right to define their own gender identity. Trans people should be recognized and treated as the gender they live in, whether or not they have undergone surgery, or their identity documents are up to date.

50% of trans people in Ontario earn less than $15000/year, despite the fact that over 70% have completed at least some college or university education.

Only 37% have succeeded in obtaining full-time employment. Being trans makes it difficult for workers to obtain letters of reference and academic transcripts.

Facts:

A study in Manitoba and Northwestern Ontario revealed that 28% of transgender have attempted suicide at least once.

Approximately 5% of the population is Transgender.

10% of the Transgender population has reported to attempt to commit suicide .

Transgenders are 2X's more likely to think about attempting suicide than Gay, Lesbian or Bisexual.

22% - 43 % of all Transgenders have attempted suicide in their life time.

2/3 of trans youth report recent self harm within the previous year.

49% of trans students, 33% of lesbian students and 40% of gay male students have experienced sexual harassment in school in the last year (2011).

It is estimated that about 0.005% to **0.014**% of people assigned male at birth and 0.002% to **0.003**% of people assigned female at birth would be diagnosed with gender dysphoria, based on 2013 diagnostic criteria, though this is considered a modest underestimate.

Thank You! to all my family and friends that have supported me through this incredible journey.
Sometimes this journey took me to places that I didn't want to go!
But in the end, I got to be the person I always knew I was.
I could not have done this without help from the Family Health Team, my Doctor, the surgeons, therapist and more.
But most of all I could not have done this without the wonderful support of my sons, my parents, my family and all of the wonderful friends and fellow employees, and employer, for hearing my voice.

Jennifer Edrei Brown

Don't suffer like I did for many years,
Speak up and be heard!
Roar! and Roar! the loudest you ever have.
Stand up, and be heard, be seen,
And live!

Be the person you were born to be!

Be proud to be born part of PRIDE,
Not everyone in life gets to be part of a group so strong and brave and fearless.

Today is your Day!
Be the Lion or Lioness you want to be!

My Mother has written several

Children's books,

in a series called:

A SPECIAL PLACE IN MY HEART!

A Place,

I Never Felt I Had Before,

But It Was There All This Time!

I Just Didn't See It!.

I Love You Mom and Dad,

and my Brother and Sister-in law and their children.

Also my two sons for standing not in front of me,
nor beside me,

but

Behind me all the way!

I dedicate this book to my Son, whom so bravely decided to take on the world by himself, ready or not.

He could have made a choice to live his life with deep depression or worse.

He chose to raise his children by himself. Thus making it that much harder to protect and care for his 2 sons, yet at the same time holding all of his own emotions inside for no one to see. Suffering more and more each day. Even with all of the mixed up feelings that he was having, he knew that he had to stay brave enough, and strong enough to make sure both boys themselves would one day understand and support his new journey.

They are what he lives for!
We love you Jennifer Endrei Brown,
Where have you been hiding!
It's time to come home!

Love Mom and Dad.

FROM LION TO LIONESS

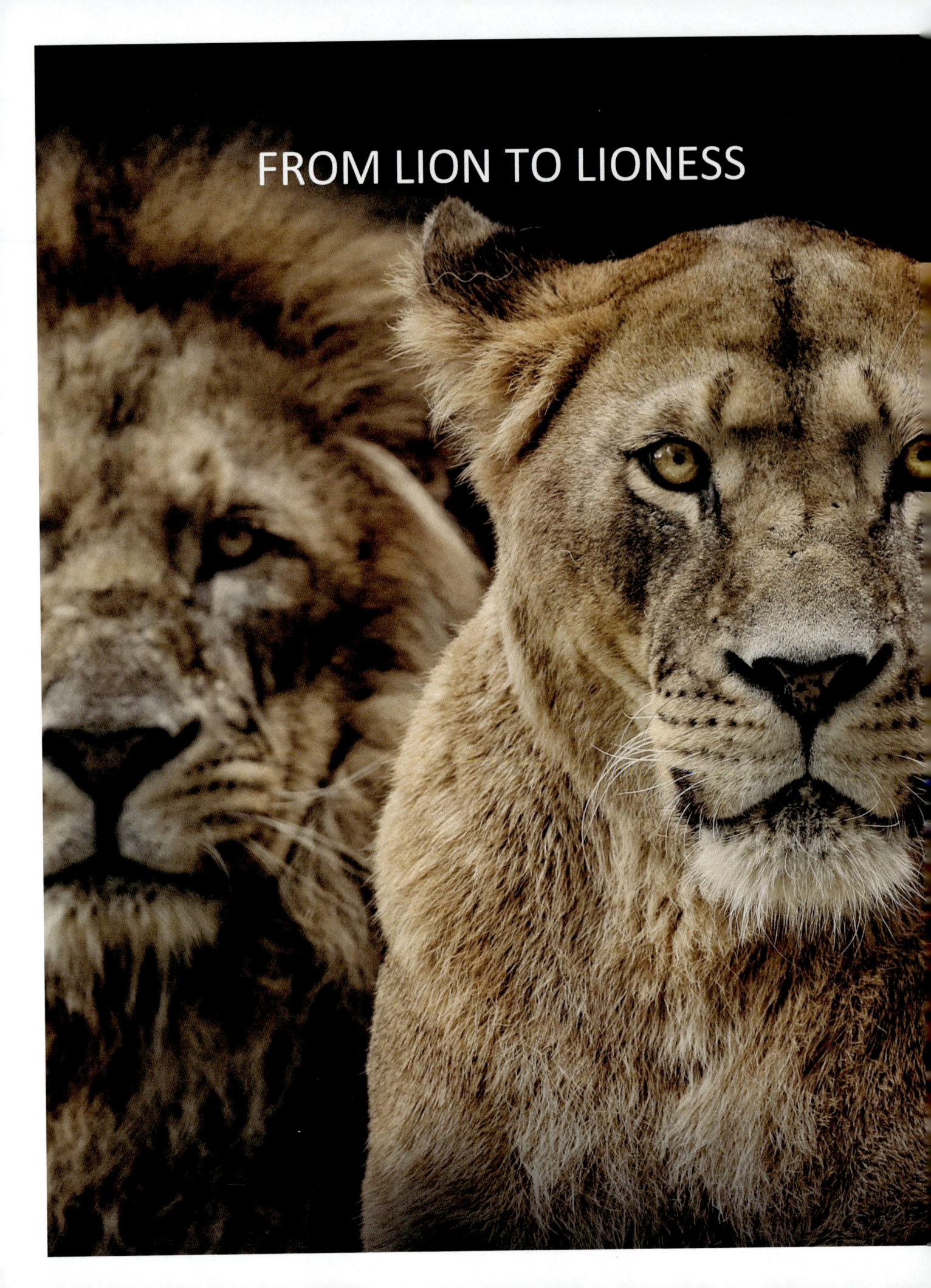

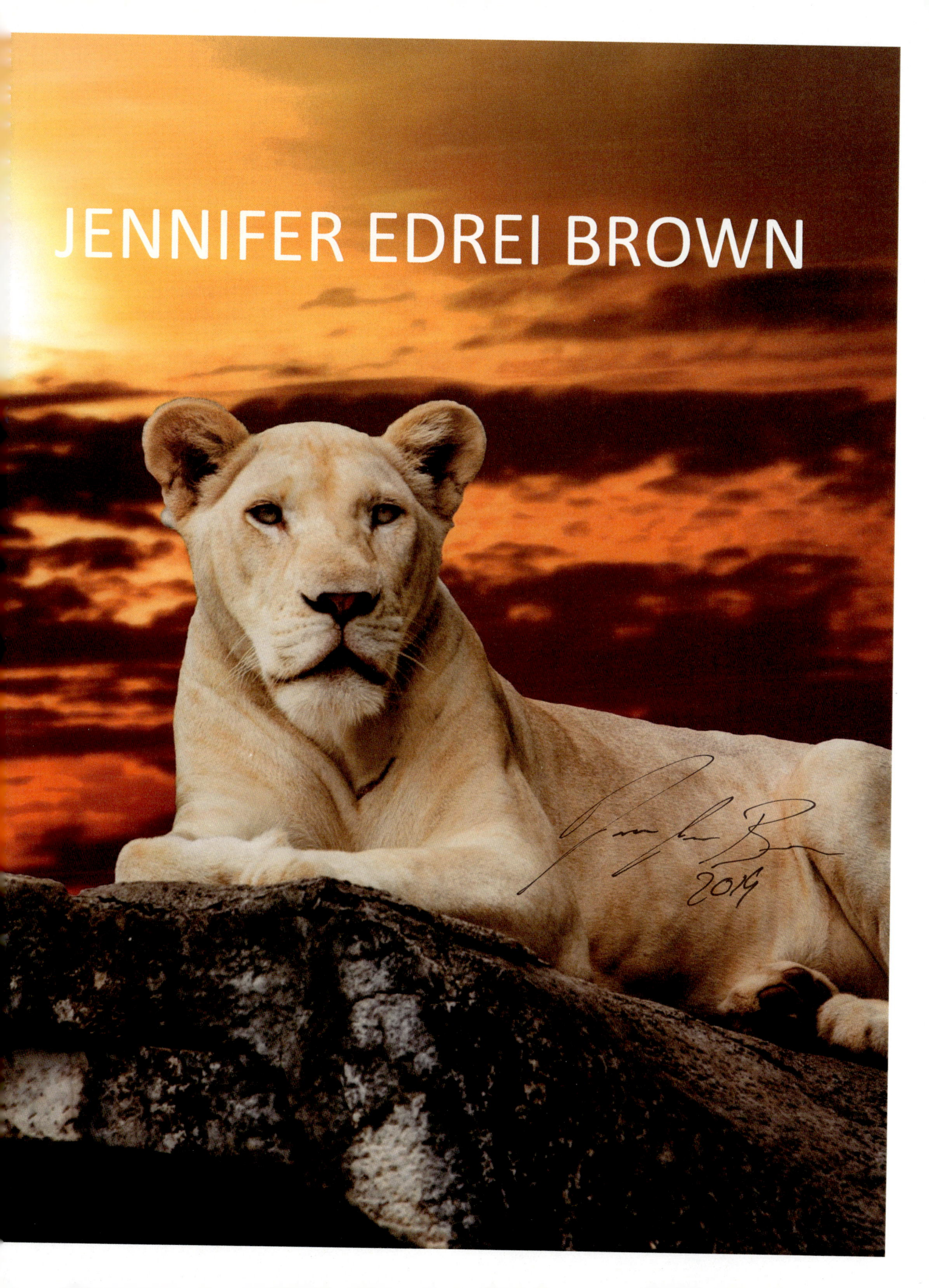

JENNIFER EDREI BROWN

No one cares
about the shape of a peanut
when they break open the shell.
They just all love,
the peanut inside!

Elisabeth Brown 2019.